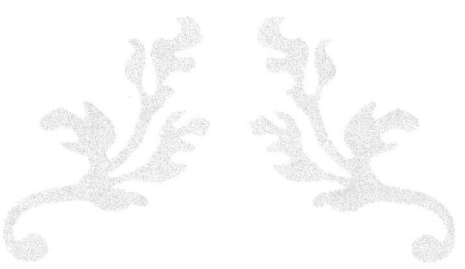

Jittery Baby

The Mimics of Fits in Early Infancy

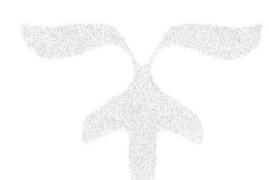

By

Renuka Chatterjee

Disclaimer

The book, "Jittery Baby & The Mimics of Fits in Infancy", is not a substitute for medical consultation. The medical information provided here is only for the purpose of awareness.

The matter in the book is a general explanation for involuntary movements perceived during early infancy. It is not to be used for or relied upon for any diagnostic or treatment purposes. The information gathered needs to be applied individually for correct interpretation. Examination of the baby by a doctor can never be substituted.

Although I have made every effort to ensure that the information in this book is all correct, I disclaim responsibility and shall have no liability, for any damages, loss, injury, or liability whatsoever suffered as a result of your reliance on the information contained in this book.

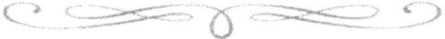

Dedicated

To

Infants & Their Parents

Preface

Usually, the jitters of having the baby have hardly subsided when anxious parents notice jittery movements in their newborn. The anxiety shoots up. Elders and the friends who are parents of more mature children reassure the young couple, but with little success. The thoughts "are my baby's brain and nerves normal" haunts the new parents. After all, they have often heard of abnormal involuntary movements being associated with severe neurological issues. They disregard the reassurances and decide to visit their doctor.

Anxious parents are barely able to bring together their concern in a proper set of words. They mumble to the doctor, "is my baby alright doc? She has tremors even when she is asleep." The doctor quickly comprehends the problem, and discharges them with a statement, "oh, it is normal for newborns. Don't worry, all will be fine as the baby grows". The doctor thinks she has done her bit.

Parents leave the clinic, but their questions are not answered. On the contrary, more are added, "did doctor mean all is not well now"? Is my baby's brain not fully formed yet? – and so on. This book is an answer to many such questions that torment the parents.

The book is meant to create awareness, not to scare

It is crucial to identify innocent developmental movement disorders in infants. They are characterized by the absence of associated neurological signs and by their favorable outcome. Nevertheless, developmental deviations have been noted in some of the affected children.

The underlying mechanisms of "innocent developmental movement disorders of infancy" are generally unknown. Most are believed to be related to subtle modifications of brain maturation. Some however may represent age-

dependent signs of a variety of disorders affecting immature neuronal networks.

Adequate scientific knowledge on the subject can prevent unnecessary concern, needless costly investigations, and ineffective and potentially toxic treatments. Too much of medical information can at times get nerve racking. The key is not to ignore that which arouses your concern.

Seek expert opinion

The book is not a substitute for proper medical consultation. Evaluation of the case by a doctor can never be over emphasized.

The mimics of fits in infancy are mainly identified on the basis of clinical examination, medical history, and of course detailed objective description of the paroxysmal episodes. But parents are often at a loss to describe distressing periodic attacks of their baby without mingling the narration with their feelings and opinions. *Video recordings of the abnormal movements can, therefore, be a great asset.*

Please do not chase all possible causes of abnormal movements during infancy that are mentioned in this book. If your observations are not associated with corroborative neurological findings, the doctor will obviously pass them off as "signs of no consequence".

Trust the doctor you choose

One good opinion is as good as ten. Regular follow-ups with the same doctor till the baby is up and about on her feet would be more fruitful than having several new consultations at different points of childhood development.

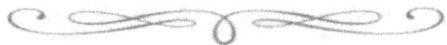

Contents

Section III - Rare Causes

Appendix

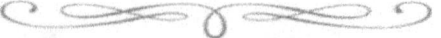

Illustrations

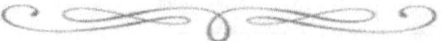

Acknowledgements

No one can accomplish a book without the inputs from the environment,
Nor have I.
Unabating encouragement from my friends and family made it possible,
especially that of my husband, Anup Chatterjee.

I owe it
To the visitors to my website, who wished to know much more on
"Abnormal Movements in Infancy" than the pages on
"Newborn Jitteriness, Twitching and Seizures" could contain.
To the Library to let me dig out the literature
that was so very essential for this book.

I an immensely grateful
To numerous websites for leaving lines of hope and tips
for those who are new to publishing a book.
To Create Space, Amazon, and Kindle to make it happen.

Lastly
To my dear dog Glo,
Who, in spite of his puppyhood, curtailed his naughtiness
and put on his best behaviour to give me time to finish the book.
Besides, he was always there to take me out in the fresh air to unwind my
entangled thoughts.

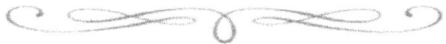

Introduction

Abrupt involuntary jitters in young infants are the common cause of concern. Most of them are consistent with normal neurological functioning for the age and the emotional state of infants, but some may represent a red flag for an underlying disorder that needs prompt attention.

Both neglect and hysterical reaction to repeated episodes of seizure-like activity give rise to several social, psychological and health issues. It is, therefore, wise to take an early consultation to eliminate treatable causes of paroxysmal movement disorders in infancy.

Indeed, jitteriness can sometimes be a clinical sign of an underlying disorder; depending on its severity, age of onset, and the associated clinical findings. This book imparts precisely this knowledge. Awareness of a variety of mimics of fits would surely help parents seek a rational approach towards a situation that steals their joy.

Most paroxysmal motor phenomena during early infancy are an innocent outcomes of an imbalance of impulse transmission through the developing nervous system. This, however, does not negate the need for essential medical attention. On the contrary, a regular evaluation of the child's development is crucial for an early diagnosis and timely intervention; more so in cases of rare neurological and non-neurological causes of jitteriness.

The book, "Jittery Baby & the Mimics of Fits in Infancy", is neither a handbook for diagnosis nor for the management of such cases. It describes various fit like activities commonly noted during early infancy, and how they get affected by a baby's pattern of behaviour and sleep. It also brings about the understanding that many clinical conditions other than brain injury could present with recurrent involuntary movements. These in turn could influence the normal behaviour of the affected infant. In short, the focus herein is to answer the range of questions that torment young parents of infants with jitteriness.

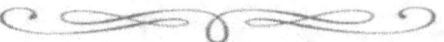

Section I
Jitteriness in Newborns

1. A Frightening Sight

It was the evening of my first day "on call" after my senior colleagues had left when a ward assistant came running up to me in panic. He forwarded a note from the nurse and said that I must go with him immediately. The nurse from the postnatal ward had written, "baby is doing something under the blanket, come at once."

Doing something under the blanket? I mumbled. What could a newborn baby do, and that too under the blanket? Well, newborns are all the time under the blanket, so maybe. I was confused. There was no time to ask anyone. I ran.

On reaching, I found a junior midwife caring for the baby. She was waiting for me at the side of the patient's bed. She looked pale and anxious. Both, the baby and the mother were fast asleep – under the blanket, of course. Just as I took a breath of relief, the nurse murmured, "Is the baby ok Doc? She is not moving now! " Not moving? What does that mean? My heart missed few beats.

I gathered courage and advanced to examine the baby. This amounted to disturbing the comforting sleep of the mother and her child, who were just trying to recover from the distress of normal childbirth. But I had no choice. Examine her I must. I woke up the mother to take permission to examine her young one. That got her started. "Is something wrong with my baby? Doctor tell me honestly what is wrong", she blurted.

My nervousness and ignorance were no less than hers. However, I reassured her and picked the baby for examination. As I touched the baby her little hands started trembling. The nurse brightened up and said, "yes doc, this is what she has been doing. See her feet are also trembling."

I shifted my gaze towards the baby's feet. I couldn't quite see the feet because of the blanket, but noticed the mother weeping. Close to my chest and firmly secure in my arms, I marked baby's tremors disappear. But they returned instantly on placing the baby on the examination table.

I examined. Her colour was good, and eyes were bright. Breathing was normal. Movements and reflexes were robust. As I laid the stethoscope on her chest, the jitteriness reappeared, but her heart was beating rhythmically.

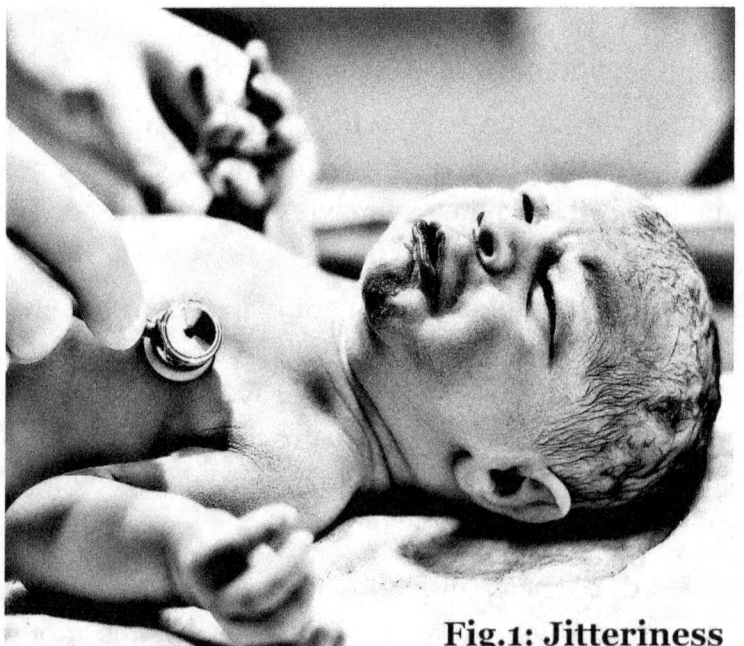

Fig.1: Jitteriness
The Startled, Crying And Distressed Neonates Are Jittery

The tremors appeared and disappeared as and when the baby felt disturbed; either due to my handling her, or by loud sound. I took a sigh of relief, and confidently reassured the mother, "it is the normal jitteriness of a newborn baby, which usually last for 72 hours after birth. In some babies they may persist for a week or 10 days, but generally not beyond 2 weeks of life, especially when there have been no complications at or before birth.

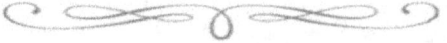

2. Normal Jitteriness of Newborns

The tiny trembling fingers of a newborn send a wave of fear through the parents. Most babies are jittery during the first few days of life. These innocent involuntary movements in neonates are commonly known as jitteriness, which has several synonyms like tremulousness, shivering, jerkiness, quivering, trembling, and shuddering. Moreover, the term jitteriness is often used rather unselectively for all forms of recurrent unusual and unintended muscular activity noted in infants.

The hallmark of jitteriness is impulsive symmetrical trembling of the limbs of both the sides in a normal full term newborn baby. The tremors are typically uniform brisk oscillations about a joint axis. They are of low amplitude and high frequency (more than 6 cycles per second), with both phases of movements being equal in speed and an amplitude of less than 3 cm. They are usually seen during spontaneous movements, and when a baby is drowsy or is being handled.

In infants "the state of the mind" (Fig. 2) influences the functions of their nervous system. Therefore, the calm and collected babies are seldom jittery, whereas those who are not quite at ease are

frequently tremulous.

In short, it is usually the startled, crying, or distressed babies who are jittery. Tremors can be easily triggered in them by external stimuli like touch or loud sounds. They can be equally easily stopped by removing the offending cause, relaxing the affected limbs by gentle flexion, or just by a reassuring touch, such as holding the limb firmly yet tenderly.

Jitteriness can advance into a clonus

At times, especially when a baby is excited, the tremulousness may advance into a clonus, another form of hyperexcitability, wherein series of involuntary, rhythmic, muscular contractions and relaxation occur in rapid succession. The coarse tremors of clonus are commonly seen at the ankle, wrist, and jaw. They are quite common in infants below 3 months of age.

Clonus commonly indicates impaired corticospinal tracts (Fig. 7) function. In young infants it is due to the immaturity of the system rather than a disease state. – More under Ankle Clonus in Infancy, pg. 34.

Differentiating normal jitteriness from the abnormal

In the absence of nervous system injury, tremulous babies neither have unusual tightness of muscles, nor altered state of alertness. Their eye movements and gaze are normal, which remain unaffected even during the episodes of jitteriness. Breathing and blood circulation irregularities, that are usually seen during fits, are never associated with normal jitteriness of early infancy.

Yet most parents associate jitteriness with fits, the common sign of a neurological disorder. The following two simple tests will help them distinguish "normal jitteriness of newborns" from a disease state causing convulsions.

1. Suckling stimulation test: Herein a jittery infant, when lying comfortably on the back with head straight and both hands left free, ceases to be tremulous as the mother places her finger in the baby's mouth, and reverts on removal of the finger.

2. Gentle bending of the affected limb or just holding it firmly and reassuringly should stop jittery movements in normal babies.

On the other hand, tremors associated with an underlying disorder persist despite initiating baby's sucking action, and also on holding the trembling limb reassuringly.

In the absence of the risk factors associated with birth process and pregnancy, mild jitteriness during first two weeks of life in an otherwise healthy baby is of no significance and can be safely ignored.

A part of normal developmental phenomena

Normal jitteriness of newborns is believed to be related to the maturation process of transmission of signals between the central & the peripheral nervous system. It is an extension of an oversensitive infantile startle response, the Moro's reflex.

Immaturity of spinal inhibitory interneurons* leads to exaggerated muscle stretch reflex (Fig. 8) which results in tremors in newborns. Moreover, jittery newborns have a high level of norepinephrine as a part of the adaptation process to extrauterine life.

Thus tremulousness of the limbs, and at times also of the chin, is the commonest involuntary movement seen during the first two weeks of life of healthy full-term newborns. It decreases as their nervous system matures. In some cases it may persist well beyond the neonatal** period, but ceases by 6 weeks of age. And by 3 years of age, most of them show normal intelligence and skills development.

Jittery babies are difficult to console

Babies when jittery, are visually inattentive, and emotionally unresponsive. Calming them becomes difficult. This causes considerable distress to the young parents. Their ability to nurture the baby suffers. Effective interaction between the parent and the baby gets more and more difficult. It hinders bonding, and jeopardizes the development of the child. Appropriate visual attention for age is crucial for the healthy acquisition of skills.

Parents should therefore seek early guidance

At times jitteriness can indeed be a clinical sign of an underlying disorder, depending on its severity, time of appearance and associated findings.

***Interneuron:** Neuron between the primary sensory neuron and the final motor neuron (Fig. 8). It is a sort of a "circuit breaker" in the nervous system.

****Neonatal:** Relating to the period from birth to the first 28 days of life.

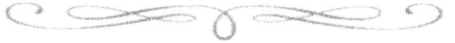

3. Behaviour Pattern of Jittery Neonate

Neonates' "state of mind" is divided into only two broad categories, asleep and awake. Even then, there is a distinct individuality in their behaviour, particularly in those who are fully mature at birth. Their response to inputs from the environment is influenced by their state of alertness, reaction to stress, and capacity for self-regulation*.

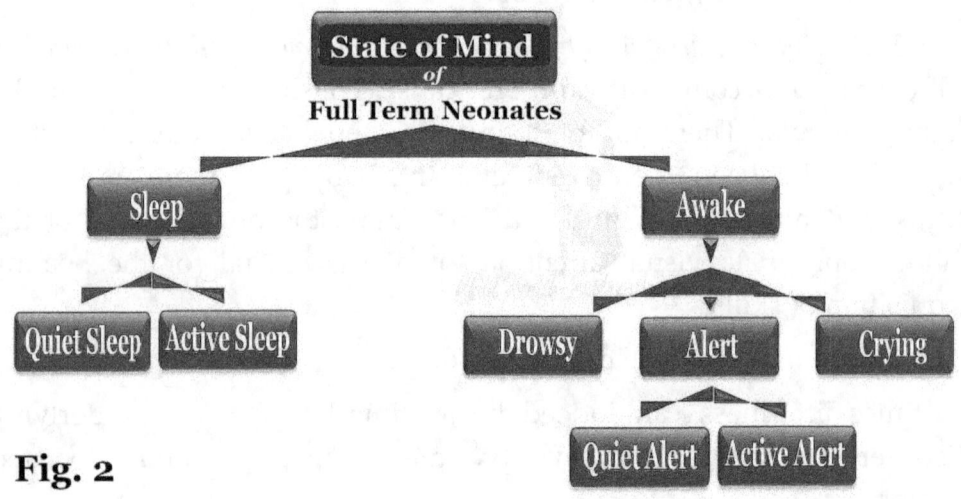

Fig. 2

Infants change their state of mind to achieve a suitable response to their needs and surroundings. They qualify a stimulus as appropriate or inappropriate, and accordingly they themselves regulate their behaviour. Following are the behaviours of significance associated with different states of an infant's mind.

- Posture
- Type of body activity
- Gaze
- Eye movements

- Facial expressions
- Breathing pattern
- Response to stimulation and personal needs

Behaviour varies with degree of self-regulation

Self-regulation is a learnt process. Babies who are nurtured with affection and care develop good self-control from early days of life. But affection is never instant, and the needs of the newborns are urgent, continuous, and often unclear. This makes parenting them a great challenge, more so for the restless inconsolable jittery infants. *The development of self-regulation in jittery babies therefore suffers a serious setback.*

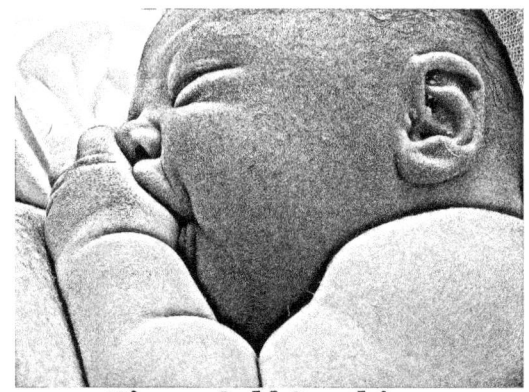

Fig. 3: Self-Soothing
Thumb Sucking
A Common Way Babies Calm Themselves

Self-regulation starts soon after birth, when it is mainly involved with consolability, sleep and feeding pattern of the baby. The level of its development in the first month of life predicts the child's future cognitive abilities, which is the core of intelligence and social success.

Effect of mother's emotional health

Babies born to mothers who suffered from stress, depression or anxiety during pregnancy are more prone to jitteriness. The development of their nervous system network gets compromised. The functional relationship between their nervous system and their hormone system is hindered. Together they cause increased excitability and restlessness, and so the jittery behaviour in these infants. Their EEG** shows asymmetric waves on the frontal region of the brain (Fig. 4) The irregular heartbeats, noticed in some of these infants is attributed to the impaired function of Vagus nerve, the 10th cranial nerve.

----

* **Self-regulation:** It is the ability to focus attention, control emotions, delay gratification and suppress impulsive behaviours such as crying. Infants with good self -regulatory skills can be easily consoled.

Electroencephalography (EEG): It is the record of the electrical activity in different parts of the brain on paper or on an oscilloscope screen. It is used to evaluate various types of brain disorders, most commonly a seizure. Others being tumours, long-term difficulties with thinking or memory, muscle weakness associated with a stroke, etc.

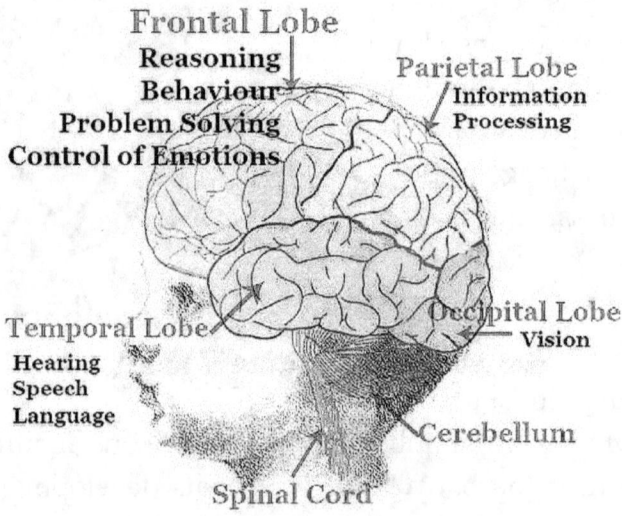

Fig. 4: Lobes of the Brain

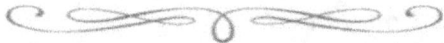

4. *Predisposing Factors of Jitteriness*

<u>In the mother</u>

Medical:

1. Depression
2. Diabetes
3. High Blood Pressure
4. Pre-eclampsia
5. Prolonged Second Stage of Labour
6. Medications
7. Autoimmune Hyperthyroidism (Grave's Disease)

Lifestyle:

1. Stress
2. Irregular or long working hours
3. Demanding social life
4. Excessive Caffeine Intake
5. Secondhand Tobacco Smoke
6. Alcohol Consumption

Addictions:

1. Chocolates
2. Coffee and other caffeine containing drinks and foods
3. Tobacco (Chewing or Smoking)
4. Alcohol
5. Recreational drugs use

In the baby

1. Deficient oxygen supply to the baby's brain during birth
2. Hypothermia: Abnormally low body temperature.
3. Prematurity
4. Low birth weight
5. Large for gestational age:

   Birth weights greater than the 97th percentile

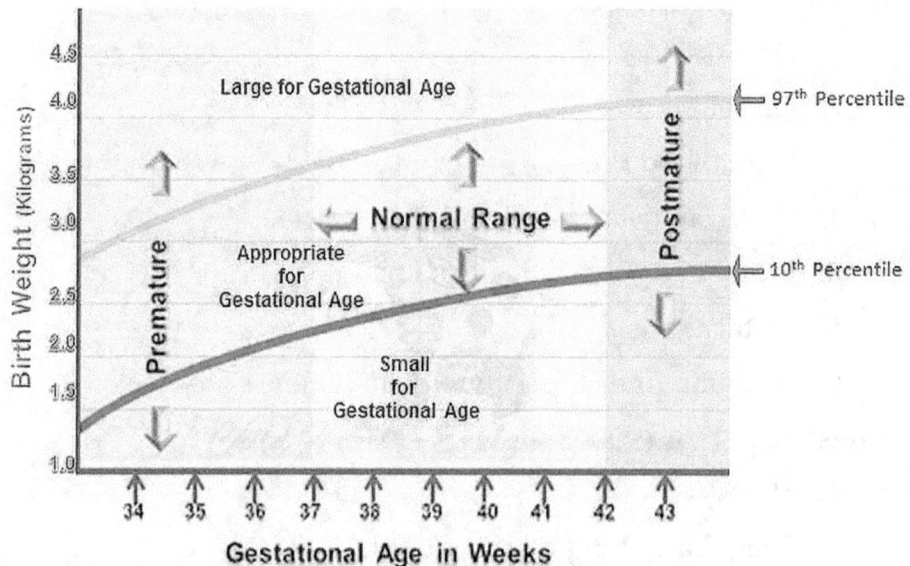

Fig. 5: **Defining Newborn Babies'**
Maturity and Appropriate Weight for Gestational Age

6. Small for gestational age;

   Weight below the 10th percentile for the gestational age.
7. Infant of diabetic mother
8. Metabolic disorders
9. Hypoglycaemia; low blood sugar
10. Hypocalcaemia; low serum calcium
11. Hypomagnesemia; low serum magnesium
12. Thyrotoxicosis, caused by over activity of the thyroid gland.

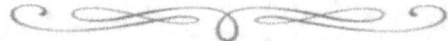

5. When Is Jitteriness Abnormal?

Jitteriness that is persistent and/or exaggerated is generally a manifestation of an underlying disorder. "Coarse" tremors are probably more often abnormal than the "fine" tremors. They seem to bear some relationship to development of choreiform* movement disorder, which is usually first noticed at school as irregular behaviour of the child.

Fine tremors

Fine tremors, when excessive, are a sign of hyperexcitability. Typically it is a withdrawal symptom in babies whose supply of stimulants from the mother is abruptly cut off at birth. Even the common dietary stimulants like coffee and chocolates, when consumed by mother in large quantities, can cause withdrawal syndrome in her newborn.

Babies of mothers who are caffeine dependent or chocoholic commonly present with hyperexcitability syndrome; unrestrained fine tremors, irritability, shrill inconsolable crying, muscular spasms, and brisk reflexes. But most of them remarkably escape developmental delays and behavioural disorders.

In contrast, *babies born of mothers who indulge in recreational drugs, alcohol or tobacco during pregnancy, are victims of abnormal growth and development, in addition to the fits due to withdrawal of the substance.* The addictive substances consumed disturb the formation of the brain of the foetus. They alter chemical messengers of the nervous system and their receptors. Consequently, these babies suffer from a variety of social and intellectual problems.

Common causes of abnormal jitteriness

1. Toxin-induced encephalopathies**
2. Mild deprivation of oxygen in the womb or during the birth process

3. Drug withdrawal***

   a.) Babies of the mothers who indulge in recreational substances such as marijuana, cocaine, opiates and the like.

   b.) Mothers on medications like selective serotonin reuptake inhibitors (SSRIs) prescribed for depression during pregnancy

4. Low blood sugar

5. Low blood calcium

6. Brain bleeds or bleeding within the skull but outside the brain

7. Mild hypothermia, fall of body core temperature below 36.5 °C

8. Poor growth in the womb (Fig. 5)

Almost all the causes listed above are due to injury to the baby in the womb, during the birth process or soon thereafter. The mild cases often go unnoticed. Moreover, it is the nature and treatability of the injury, rather than the tremor itself, that determines the ultimate likely course of the disease.

Outcome

Jittery neonates with a history of perinatal**** complications are at 30% risk of impaired learning process and skills development, particularly those with coarse tremors.

Should there be no significant perinatal history, and the tremors are coarse which do not resolve with soothing, there could be an underlying problem. In such cases the treating doctor would consider septic and metabolic screening, brain imaging, and thyroid function evaluation. *Since excessive tremulousness is a known presentation of withdrawal syndrome, the drugs taken by the mother during pregnancy would also be ascertained.*

Choreiform Movement Disorder: It comprises of brief, abrupt and irregular movements that commonly accompany the purposeful movements, and subside during sleep. The unpredictable muscle contractions have no particular pattern or distribution. They can affect any part of the body. The untimely uncontrolled jerky movements distort the manner of walking, talking, eating and all.

The affected children are unable to carry themselves well. Nor are they able to accomplish their day to day activities smoothly. They are frequently looked upon as clumsy, fidgety and ill behaved. The condition gets worse when they are worried, fearful or disturbed.

** **Toxin-induced Encephalopathy**: Encephalopathy is a disease of the brain wherein its functions are adversely affected by some agent or condition such as viral infection, toxins in the blood, or electrolytes and hormones imbalance.

*** **Drug withdrawal:** In neonates this implies that at birth their supply of the drugs from the mother's blood is abruptly cut off.

******Perinatal:** Childbirth related, which could be at birth, or anytime during the period extending approximately from the 28th week of gestation to the 28th day after birth.

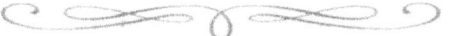

6. Chin Tremors

During the initial days of life, almost all normal newborns periodically get spontaneous tremors of the chin, particularly when they are cold, crying, or under stress. It is more common in babies who are born preterm, also among those who are exposed to second-hand tobacco smoke either before or after birth, or both.

The precise functional deviation, if any in these babies, yet remains unclear. Their neurological development is noted to be overall normal. Therefore, like most of the other mimickers of seizure disorders in infancy, chin tremors are also attributed to the immaturity of the nervous system.

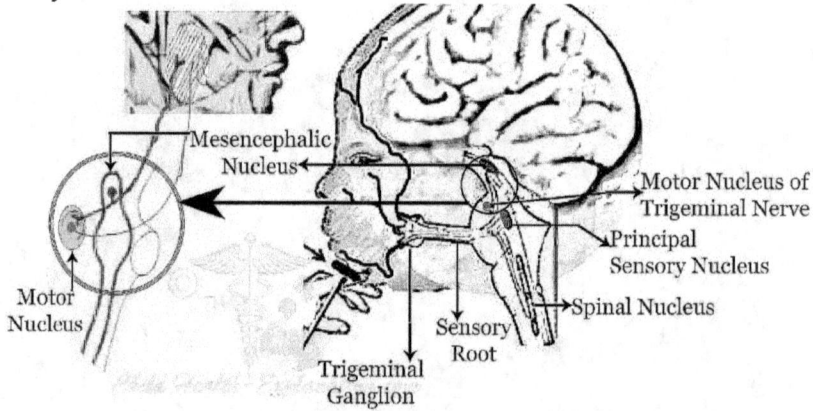

Fig. 6: Jaw Jerk - A Single Synapse Stretch Reflex

Unrestrained jaw jerk

Jaw-jerk, like other deep tendon reflexes, is used to access the integrity of the neuromuscular pathway; in this case that of the trigeminal nerve*. Underdeveloped spinal inhibitory interneurons (Fig. 8) of young infants are unable to restrain the stretch reflex in their muscles. As a result, sudden opening of the mouth sets in rhythmic contractions of the jaw muscles, perceived as trembling chin. In normal babies, the tendency of chin tremors wanes off as they mature. *But if it persists* *beyond 3 months of age it could indicate forthcoming developmental issues, especially in a baby who has associated neurological signs or history of perinatal complications.*

Causes of chin tremors

The bilaterally symmetrical tremulousness of jaw suggests that the abnormality could either lie within the muscle itself or be an effect of perinatal injury to the higher nervous system. Hypoxic ischemic encephalopathy and intracranial bleed are the two most common causes of brain injury in neonates. Even so, only about one-third of the babies with birth related difficulties develop disabilities. All don't.

The effect at muscles level may be seen in following conditions:
In the baby:
1. Cold stress
2. Low blood sugar levels
3. Calcium-magnesium imbalance
4. Transient hyperthyroidism secondary to Graves' disease in the mother.
5. Hereditary chin tremors, a rare autosomal dominant (Fig. 25) condition linked to chromosome 9q13-21 – more on pg. 80.

In mother:
1. Tobacco smoke
2. Alcohol consumption
3. Excessive intake of caffeine containing drinks
4. Use of recreational drugs during pregnancy

Medical evaluation a must

Frequent chin tremors, more so in absence of obvious distress need the doctor's attention. EEG and MRI evaluation may seem unnecessary but are the only way to clinch the underlying cause, if any.

Trigeminal Nerve (5th Cranial Nerve): Mainly the nerves of the head and the neck. It supplies sensations to the face, mucous membranes, and other structures of the head. It controls biting and chewing movements.

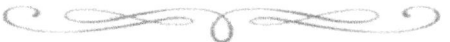

7. Ankle Clonus in Infancy

Most babies in their first 2 months of life have sporadic episodes of rhythmic back and forth movement of one or both ankles. Though each such episode lasts for only a fraction of a second, they arouse considerable concern in the parents. Internet search qualifies these steady high-speed oscillatory movements as ankle clonus, a well-known sign of nervous system dysfunction. This sends parents in frenzy of fear. More search leads to more scary causes of nervous system disorder. But, in infancy, the unsustained ankle clonus (≤5 beats/sec) is seldom a sign of nervous system damage.

What is ankle clonus?

Ankle clonus indeed indicates impairment in carrying down the commands from the brain. The injury or defect that impedes the transmission of impulses along the nerves could be at the level of the brain, spinal cord or corticospinal tracts, the complex bundles of connecting nerve fibres (Fig. 7). Thus the required movement gets converted into reflex coarse tremor like oscillatory movements, at an unwavering frequency of 5- 8 cycles per second.

Though clonus of the ankle is most widely known, in general clonus can occur in any muscle, like that of the knee cap, jaw, wrist and other muscles of arms and legs.

The mechanism of clonus in infancy remains unclear

The presence of ankle clonus during infancy is very common, but there are hardly any studies which evaluate the cause of clonus in healthy babies. This could be because it is almost impossible to justify a neurological study on normal newborns. Most of the effort is therefore driven to determine if the infant with ankle clonus has any associated neurological deficit.

Fig. 7: Pathways from the Brain to the Spinal Cord

Motor Cortex*

→ Motor Cortex*

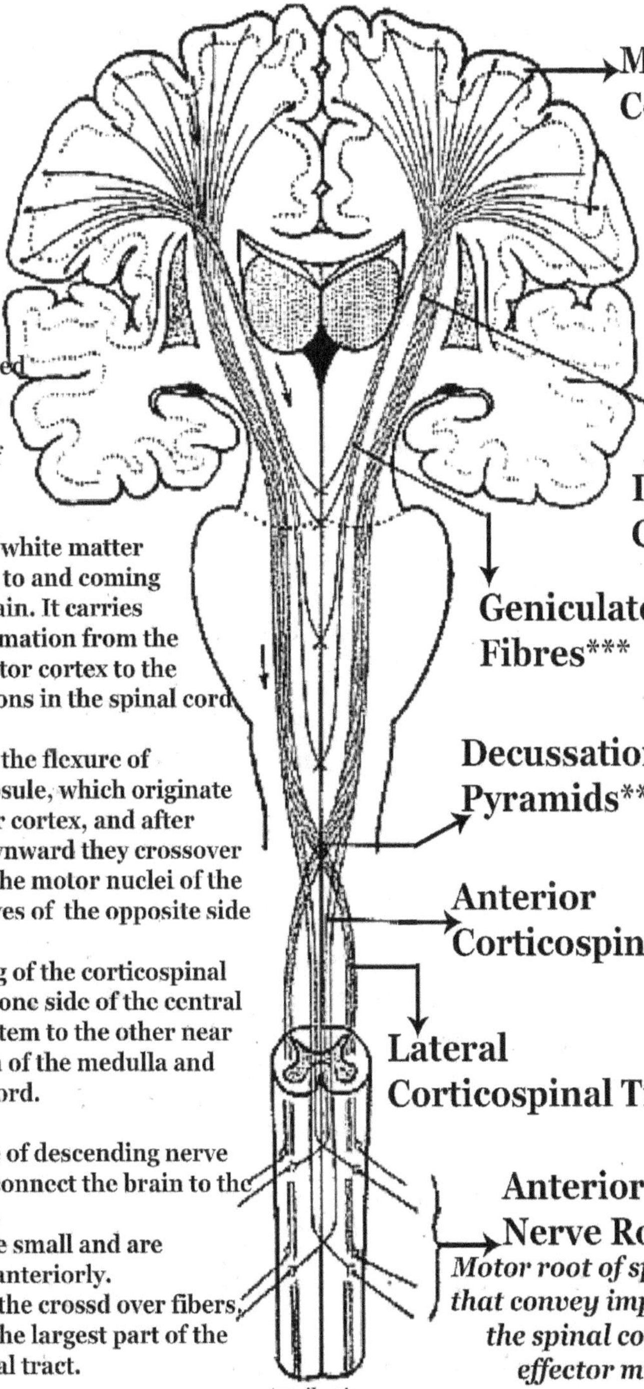

*Area of the brain involved in planning, control and execution of actions.

**Cluster of white matter fibres going to and coming from the brain. It carries motor information from the primary motor cortex to the motor neurons in the spinal cord

***Fibres at the flexure of internal capsule, which originate in the motor cortex, and after passing downward they crossover and end in the motor nuclei of the cranial nerves of the opposite side

****Crossing of the corticospinal tracts from one side of the central nervous system to the other near the junction of the medulla and the spinal cord.

*****Bundle of descending nerve fibres that connect the brain to the spinal cord.
Anterior are small and are positioned anteriorly.
Lateral are the crossd over fibers, They form the largest part of the corticospinal tract.

Internal Capsule**

Geniculate Fibres***

Decussation of Pyramids****

Anterior Corticospinal Tract

Lateral Corticospinal Tract*****

Anterior Nerve Roots
Motor root of spinal nerve that convey impulses from the spinal cord to the effector muscles

Is ankle clonus normal during infancy?

Bilateral ankle clonus of 3 to 5 beats is of no consequence, especially in those infants who are less than 6 months old and are distressed, crying, hungry, or jittery. It is the sustained ankle clonus (≥8 beats/sec) that arouses concern. But like infantile reflexes, this too could be the representation of immature neuromuscular control, which disappear gradually with the development of postural balance and coordination.

The age at which an infant begins to react aptly to the signals received through nerves is very individual. The delay in neuromuscular control development is extremely common, and it runs in families. *Therefore, in most cases, even a fairly well-sustained ankle clonus, of about 5 - 8 beats/sec, by itself is of no significance. Its importance as a neurological sign that is worthy of attention depends on an associated medical history and the clinical presentation of the case.*

Furthermore, infants while trying to achieve a comfortable posture often develop involuntary, rhythmic, oscillatory movements. If these movements involve a joint like wrist or ankle, they mimic clonus. *Therefore, the ankle and wrist clonus that are noted by parents when the baby is supposedly lying down comfortably could be the result of the baby's efforts to change the posture. A similar effect is also seen at the wrist joints when young babies are being fed; an effort to participate in the feeding process.*

How does development affect the diagnosis?

By definition, clonus is a sign of movement disorders that involve the corticospinal tract dysfunction, yet almost all normal newborns exhibit ankle clonus during the first 4 weeks of life. This is attributed to increased reactivity of their immature cortical spinal tract (Fig. 7), but then the clonus in a normal baby is never sustained.

This concludes:

1. Ankle clonus of more than ten beats any time, even during the first year of life, indicates the presence of an abnormally hyperactive stretch reflex.
2. Ankle clonus that persists beyond 3 months of age arouses suspicion of subsequent development of neurological abnormality, or postural instability.

3. *Ankle clonus beyond 6 months of age suggests impaired development of the nervous system.*

Role of stretch reflex

In neurological disorders, clonus is usually associated with hyperactive stretch reflexes (Fig. 8), where in response to a sudden change in the tension of muscle, a strong signal is transmitted to the spinal cord via the muscle spindle, which is the sensory apparatus in the belly of the muscle. This brings about an instantaneous strong reflex contraction or relaxation of the muscle from which the signal had originated.

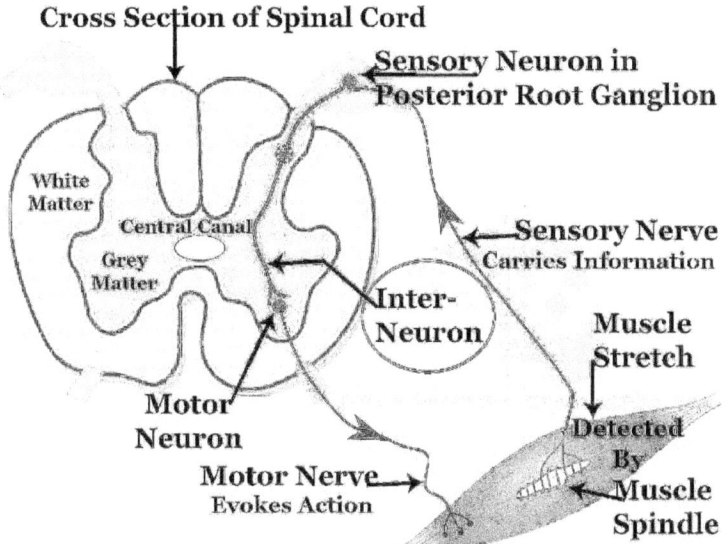

Fig. 8: Pathway of Stretch Reflex
Phenomenon that provides steady posture & coordination of movements

The normal stretch reflex provides steady posture and coordination of the movements. It forms the basis for the development of skills to perform intricate activities smoothly and efficiently. When it is compromised the actions become jerky and clumsy, as in diseases of nervous system, metabolic disorder, chemical toxins from recreational or medical drugs, or due to an underdeveloped nervous system.

Brain development is an ongoing process

Rapid brain growth that starts in the womb extends well through the third year of life. The central nervous system has a remarkable capacity to respond to the baby's needs in a dynamic manner. Inputs from the surroundings modify the circuits of the nervous system. Therefore, soon after birth the baby's brain begins to form new pathways, which connect the nerve cells and transmit the impulses appropriately. This phenomenon is called plasticity of the nervous system.

Neuroplasticity is not only the basis of a healthy and adaptive system development, but it also plays a crucial role in the recovery of the nervous system from the minor insults incurred during the birth process. Besides the quality of environmental influences, the eventual recovery, however, depends on the severity of the injury.

The following factors can jeopardize optimal development of the nervous system.

1. Maternal stress, fatigue or infection

2. Diet deficient in Vitamins, Iron, and other essential nutrients

3. Exposure to second-hand smoke

   Intrauterine and/or during early infancy

4. Irregular lifestyle of the parents

5. Family discord

6. Disturbed mental health of the parents

7. Mothers indulging in alcohol, or recreational drugs

8. Birth process related injuries

9. Metabolic disorders in the baby

10. Restricted intrauterine development:
    Whether born premature or with growth retardation, the causes that hamper a baby's development in the womb, can also jeopardize the maturation of its nervous system.

Medical opinion is necessary for the diagnosis

A tricky situation arises when the nature of clonus is equivocal, and the underlying cause is ambiguous. Disturbed parents then tend to lose faith in the doctor. But a short follow-up with one neurologist or consultations with several experts at different point of the child's development do not resolve diagnostic dilemma.

Close follow-up at regular intervals till 18 months of age is essential to arrive at a definite diagnosis. The possibility of the development of a neurologic abnormality at a later date can be ruled out only by periodic evaluation of the pattern of a child's development, more so in infants who present with a significant clonus, but without other neurologic findings.

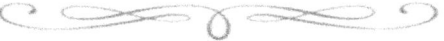

8. Tics and Twitches

The terms tics and twitches are often used interchangeably for brief involuntary actions and sounds that are rapid, repetitive, non-rhythmic, and totally out of the blue. They can be simple or complex.

Simple tics commonly involve the face, neck, and shoulders. In their simple form, they present as a meaningless jerking of a limb, shoulder shrugs, blinking, distorted facial expressions, or nodding. Complex motor tics appear purposeful activity such as jumping, skipping, touching or smelling objects or self, and grinding of the teeth particularly in sleep.

Vocal tics too can be simple (clearing the throat, grunting, and coughing) or complex, like uttering of unintelligible syllables or phrases usually in an explosive and clumsy fashion. Preschool children, who have outbursts of outright obscene language, particularly of words relating to faeces could be suffering from a rare disorder called coprolalia, found in cases of disturbed mental state, or Tourette's syndrome, an autosomal dominant disorder that normally does not present before 2 years of age.

Tics in neonates

Tics in neonates are a sudden and seemingly uncontrolled sharp pull of the face muscles. Like most other mimics of fits in infancy, these too could be attributed to ongoing nervous system development, especially when rest of the baby's behaviour seems normal.

Developmental factor

Right from birth, babies are bombarded with a variety of sensory inputs that are strange to them. Their ability to assimilate and respond to these with intelligible actions is at a primitive stage. Their movements are jerky and clumsy.

The ability to assimilate social cues, regulate emotions and organize expressivity for effective communication is a slow learning process. Their simple smiles and cries do develop into more complex expressions but often end in facial tics and twitches, particularly during early infancy. Thus the specificity of their expressions remains unclear, and the behaviour events get mistaken for seizures.

With maturation, their expressions get more organized. Over the first three years, their social cues become clear, and the spells that resemble fits but are not associated with abnormal electro-encephalography (EEG), disappear.

Nevertheless, some seizures like behavioural events, predominantly those that extend beyond the fifth year of life, could be secondary to underlying neurological disorder. Therefore, *even though most involuntary movements in early infancy are transient innocent events, it is best to get an in-depth medical evaluation for them all.*

Transient tic disorder of childhood

Social stress, insecurity, and separation anxiety have been linked to tic disorder of childhood. The usual age of onset is therefore during toddlerhood and early school years when children go through emotional turmoil. 1 in every 4 children experiences tics at some time or other, which usually wane off spontaneously. Attempts to suppress them only increases child's urge to perform them.

Emotional excitement and stress intensify tics, which may persist during sleep, and could naturally be mistaken for seizures. Stress tics can sometimes be seen during early infancy as well.

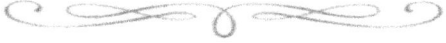

9. Shuddering Attacks

A quick shudder at the sight of desired food or an interesting toy is a common expression of eagerness among infants and toddlers. Besides excitement, embarrassment and frustration also frequently bring about a bout of the whole body trembling in infants and toddlers, for example, when peeing (pg. 44).

Body shudders are at times accompanied by a stiffening of the arms. Trembling of the chin has also been noted in some cases during these episodes, particularly in those babies who are anxious or emotionally strained. The benign shuddering attacks typically last only for a few seconds, and as soon as they end, all seems well.

Shuddering movements associated with different infantile activities usually occur in healthy babies when they are awake or eating. The parents relate them to cute expressions of their newborns. But when they shudder in sleep, or when the involuntary jerking of head, shoulder, and trunk recur several times a day, a fear of a seizure disorder naturally creeps in.

Shuddering attacks are a harmless variant of normal infant behaviour. Some believe them to be a type of benign myoclonus of early infancy. Since a family history of "essential tremors" (pg. 83) is present in most of these cases, many others consider shuddering as an early manifestation of this rare hereditary movement disorder.

Moreover, the clinical presentation of shuddering attacks can be mistaken for infantile spasms, but neither MRI nor EEG recordings during and in between the events show any abnormality. Spontaneous remission occurs as the baby matures. Some continue to get them beyond toddlerhood well through the fifth year of life. These children, however, do not experience any developmental delay or deficit. They eventually outgrow the tendency to shudder. Nevertheless, it is important to have the paediatrician and a neurologist evaluate the child to ensure nothing is amiss.

10. Pee Shivers:
Post Micturition Convulsion Syndrome

The terms "pee shivers", "shivering after urination", and "post-micturition* convulsion syndrome" are commonly comprehended as the **fit like movements** that come after the act of voiding is complete. But that is not always the case. More often than not, it is just when some urine leaks through the external sphincter (Fig. 8), the infants' little body jolts a few times. Each episode usually lasts for about 5 seconds, after which the baby is completely normal.

To parents, these momentary shudders **look like seizures. Unlike seizures,** pee shivers are neither a sign of an underlying neurological abnormality nor do they leave any sequelae. As to why shivering after urination takes place; no one really knows. The probable process can be explained as follows.

Urination in infancy is a reflex phenomenon

The urinary bladder is a stretchable bag. As the urine collects in it, its wall stretches, initially without a significant rise in its internal pressure. And when the bladder is full, the stretch receptors in bladder wall trigger off the micturition reflex that sends the message to the sacral region of the spinal cord (see the "Reflex Arc" in Fig. 8). In response, the parasympathetic sacral spinal nerves to the bladder get activated. They bring about the contraction of the bladder muscle (Detrusor Muscle) and relaxation of the internal urethral sphincter. This leads to involuntary urination; a normal process in infants and toddlers.

Sudden release of bladder pressure gives shivers

The sudden release of urine from a full bladder is associated with a sudden change in the levels of neurotransmitters**, the chemicals that bring about the transfer of the impulse to another nerve and muscle fibres. This could stir up a strange sensation that results in shivering.

Micturition Reflex-Arc & Its Higher Control System

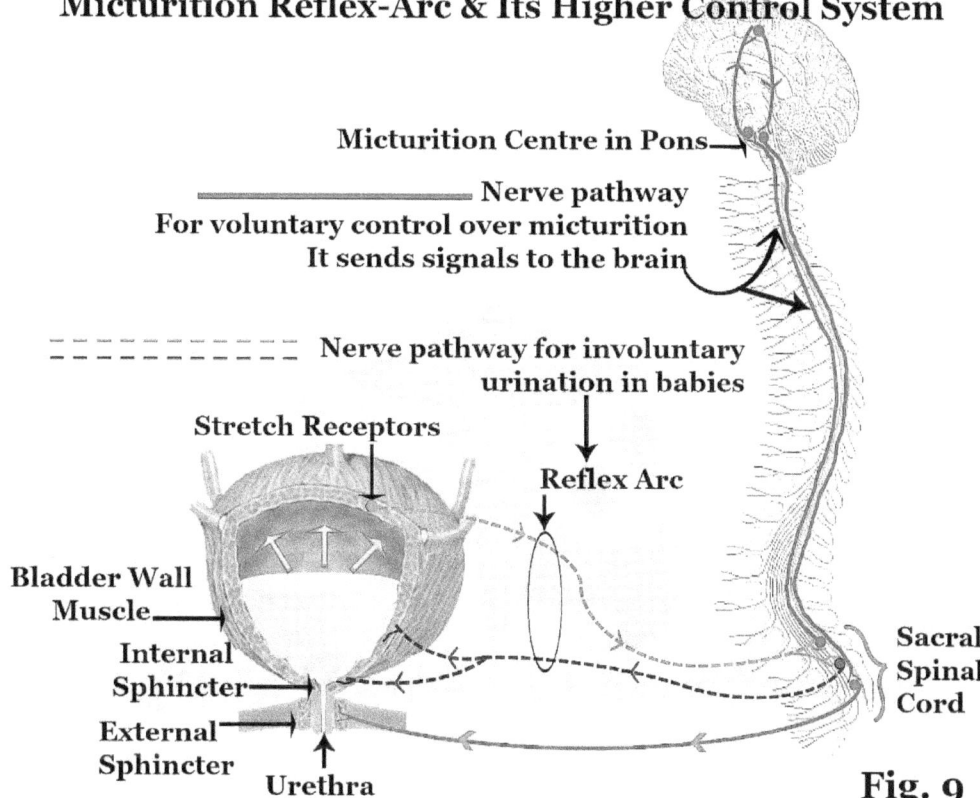

Micturition Centre in Pons

Nerve pathway
For voluntary control over micturition
It sends signals to the brain

Nerve pathway for involuntary
urination in babies

Stretch Receptors

Reflex Arc

Bladder Wall
Muscle

Internal
Sphincter

External
Sphincter

Urethra

Sacral
Spinal
Cord

Fig. 9

The force and rapidness of voiding

Intensity of shivers after urination is related to the force and rapidness of voiding. Infants void at much higher pressure, when compared to older children who have adequate control on micturition. Besides, the coordination of their bladder contractions is impaired, which causes considerable fluctuation of pressure in the bladder when they pass urine.

The fullness of the bladder

Pee shivers are believed to be directly proportional to the fullness of the bladder. Infants' bladder can hold only a small quantity of urine. When measured in millilitres, irrespective of the age of the infant, the capacity of infant's bladder is approximately 7 times the body weight in kilograms.

Not a neuro-muscular disorder

Despite the name, Post Micturition Convulsion Syndrome does not signify a movement disorder. It is also not the result of an immature nervous system. All infants do not have it. On the other hand, even adults experience it every now and then, particularly when they have to hold on for a considerable time, even though they have the urge.

In addition to the sacral spinal cord, the sensory signals from full bladder are also passed to the higher control centres in the Pons and the Cerebrum. The higher control network does awaken infants and toddlers on initiation of the reflex arc, but their voluntary control over micturition is not developed. It matures only at about 4 years of age.

----

*Micturition: The Latin word for "urination".

Neurotransmitters: A chemical switching system, which gets activated when any two nerves connect. These **chemicals are important for normal functioning of the nervous system.

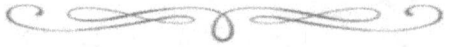

11. Neonatal Seizures Vs Jitteriness

Episodic purposeless rhythmic movements during early infancy do not always indicate nervous system impairment. The signals through an immature brain tend to overshoot. Therefore a variety of recurrent stereotyped movements that resemble fits are common during early infancy. Most parents, being unaware of the probable causes for the paroxysmal activity of their baby, fear fits, which constitute the most frequent and distinctive manifestation of neurologic disorders.

Neonatal Seizures Vs Jitteriness

Characteristic	Seizures	Jitteriness
Can External stimulus initiate?	No	Yes
Movements	Irregular and Jerky	Symmetrical Fine Tremors
Associated Rise In Heart Rate	Yes	No
Associated Breath Holding	±	No
Can Movements Be Easily Stopped?	No Self Limited Movements	Yes Gently Bending/Holding Lmb Or Making The Baby Suck

Fig. 10

The developing brain is very susceptible to seizures

Early infancy is the most vulnerable phase of life for developing seizure disorders, more so during the first few days after birth. Of 1000 babies, 1.3 to 3.5 born full term and 10 to 130 born preterm suffer symptomatic convulsions.

Neonatal seizures are seldom idiopathic*.

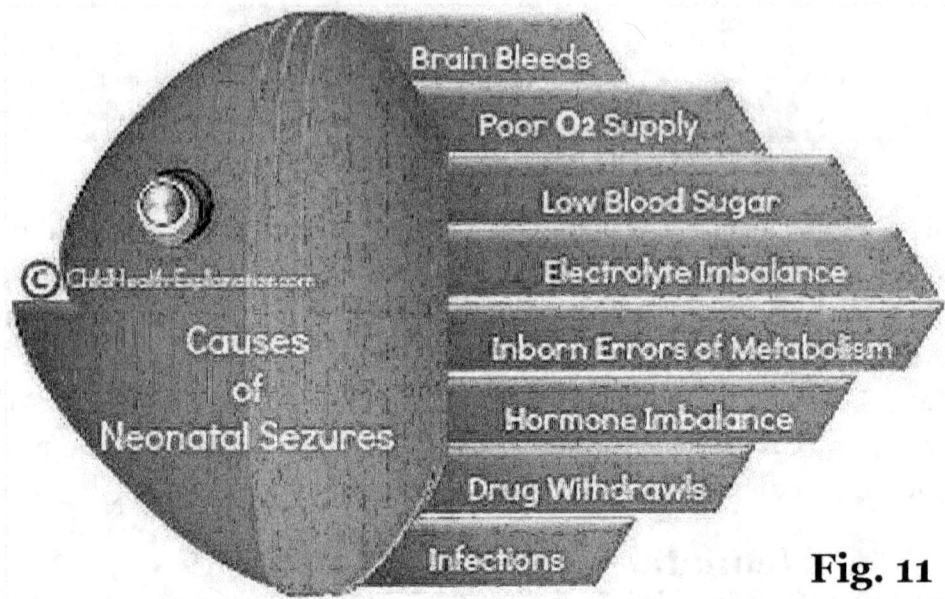

Brain Bleeds
Poor O₂ Supply
Low Blood Sugar
Electrolyte Imbalance
Inborn Errors of Metabolism
Hormone Imbalance
Drug Withdrawls
Infections

Causes of Neonatal Sezures

Fig. 11

A broad range of systemic and central nervous system disorders predispose young infants to seizure. In addition, an unfavourable environment in the womb, and circumstantial events during the birth process increase the risk of neonatal seizures (Fig. 12). The most common cause is inadequate oxygen levels, known as hypoxic-ischemic encephalopathy.

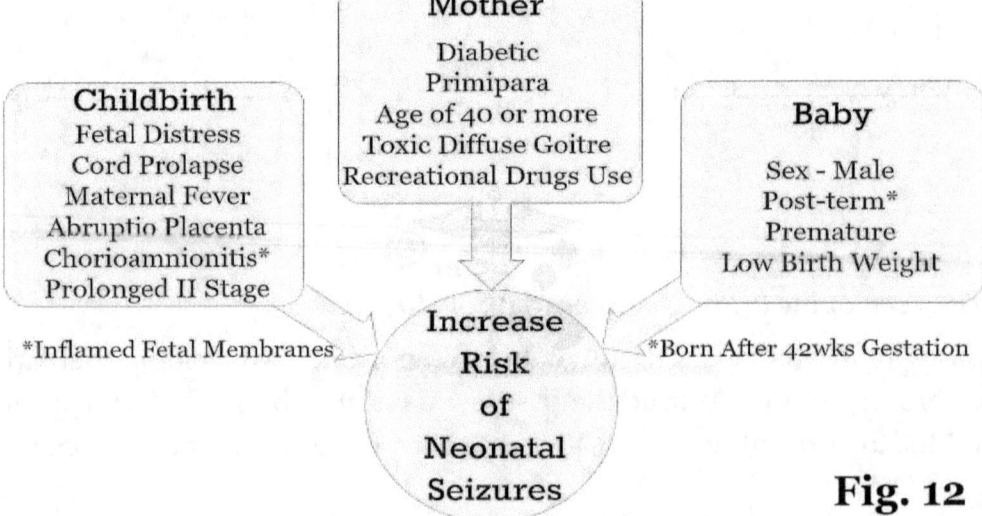

Mother
Diabetic
Primipara
Age of 40 or more
Toxic Diffuse Goitre
Recreational Drugs Use

Childbirth
Fetal Distress
Cord Prolapse
Maternal Fever
Abruptio Placenta
Chorioamnionitis*
Prolonged II Stage

Baby
Sex - Male
Post-term*
Premature
Low Birth Weight

*Inflamed Fetal Membranes

Increase Risk of Neonatal Seizures

*Born After 42wks Gestation

Fig. 12

Characteristics of neonatal seizures

Seizures are generally defined as events caused by abnormal electrical activity in the brain, some of which present as uncontrollable muscle movement and frothing. But neonatal seizures are often subtle, which can be best explained as "sudden and recurrent alterations in neurologic function". This includes the fits with and without EEG changes.

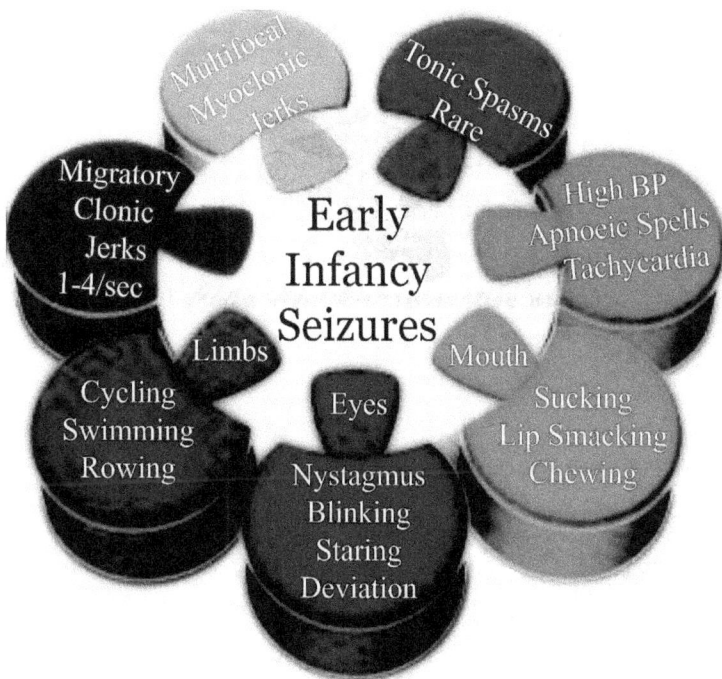

Fig. 13: Types of Neonatal Seizures

Neonatal seizures are easy to miss; some are low-key and mimic natural movements like sucking and blinking, while others are easily confused with innocent involuntary jerks of early infancy. Moreover, there is no specific diagnostic test that could pinpoint the seizures that indicate injury to the brain. Yet it is vital to distinguish the normal from abnormal.

Effect of seizures

Seizures in infancy jeopardize normal maturational processes in the developing brain. The aberrant neurogenesis and mossy fibre sprouting** is believed to increase excitability, and thereby lower the threshold for seizures. This results in long-lasting high risk for seizures, and for poor cognitive development***, emotional instability and learning disabilities in the affected children. Prompt treatment of the underlying cause and efficient control of seizures can minimize the chances of these neuro-developmental disabilities.

Difficulties in diagnosis

Only the factual description of the episodes by the parents, along with an authentic, relevant and complete perinatal history can help to reach an early diagnosis.

Clinical detection is unreliable:
Neonatal seizures are usually focal and often difficult to recognize. The sudden bursts of altered nervous system activity sets in momentary migratory clonic**** jerks of extremities, bizarre sensory perceptions, or essential organ dysfunction. During such episodes, the baby may or may not be responsive. The effective level of consciousness varies in each case.

EEG:
The abnormal electrical activity in the brain that causes seizures cannot always be ascertained on an electroencephalograph (EEG) changes. On the other hand, not all deviant recordings seen on EEG are clinically apparent fits. Despite that, the EEG is a powerful tool for the neurological diagnosis and prognosis in young infants. Those with a consistently abnormal EEG along with obvious involuntary movements would be at a risk of unfavourable neurological outcome and epilepsy.

An EEG is the gold standard for distinguishing epileptic seizures from nonepileptic paroxysmal events. It helps to detect subclinical seizure activity in high-risk babies such as perinatal hypoxic-ischemic insult and infections of the central nervous system, even in those who are already put on medications. The anticonvulsant therapy does not immediately stop abnormal electrical discharge in the brain. Initially, it only gives the symptomatic relief.

Neuroimaging:
Brain scans (Ultrasound, CT scan, and MRI) are good only to detect the structural abnormalities. Nevertheless, intracranial bleeds and tissue

damage caused by inadequate blood supply can usually be diagnosed on imaging within a few hours of injury.

For medically stable infants MRI may be the preferred form of neuroimaging, wherein determining the type and extent of the lesion is possible. It detects most brain and spinal cord malformations quite precisely. It can also identify accumulation of neuroactive chemicals associated with metabolic disorders.

----

*Idiopathic: A disease for which the cause is not known.

** Mossy Fibre Sprouting: Seizures related injury to the nerve cells within the central nervous system brings about the formation of new axon collaterals of dentate granule cells. This is called mossy fibre sprouting.

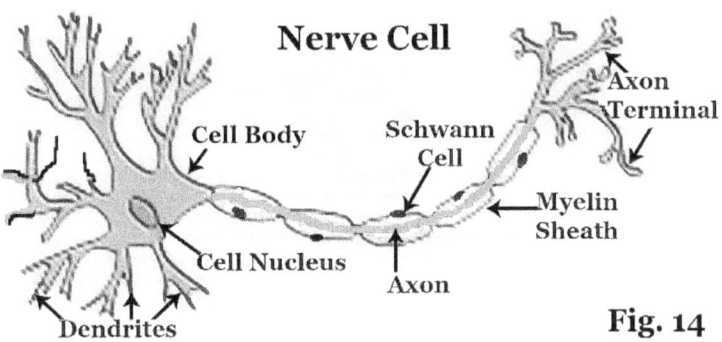

Fig. 14

***Cognitive Development: The development of intelligence; thought processing, problem-solving and decision-making ability that begins in infancy and continues through adulthood..

****Clonic: Involuntary muscular contraction and relaxation in rapid succession.

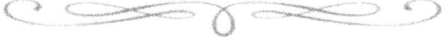

Section II
Sleep-to-Wake
Transition Disorders

12. Movements During Sleep

It is the twitching and writhing movements seen during active sleep phase of newborn babies that are commonly mistaken for fits. Contrary to the common belief, the brain is very active during sleep. Even in the absence of external inputs synchronized activity is present in the brain, particularly during Rapid Eye Movements (REM) sleep.

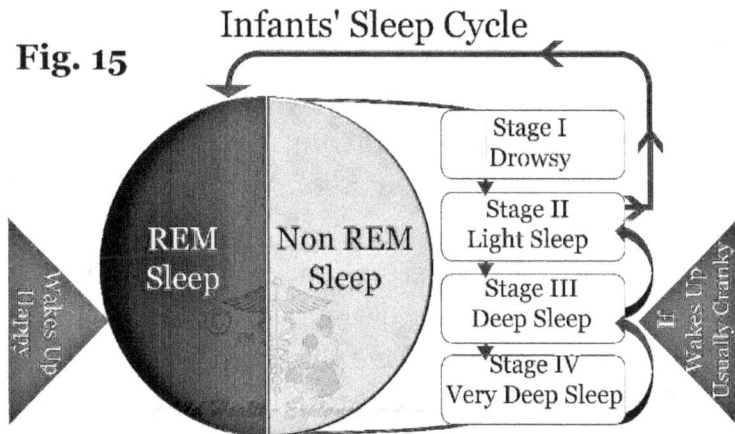

Fig. 15 — Infants' Sleep Cycle

This spontaneous continuous internal activity in the brain is believed to be necessary to retain and update information that flows in. It also helps in growth and repair of the nerve circuits according to specific needs of an individual. In short, *active sleep, also known as REM sleep, has a significant impact on overall maturation of the brain, and thereby on social, emotional, and mental development of infants*. It is therefore no wonder that the active sleep phase during infancy is 2½ times greater than that on attaining maturity.

The rest of sleep cycle is called NREM, Non Rapid Eye Movement or "quiet" sleep. This pattern of sleep helps restore energy. Low oxygen consumption and release of growth hormone during deep quiet sleep promote growth.

Babies are not easily disturbed from sleep during the deep sleep stages of NREM sleep (Fig. 15). They lie nearly still.

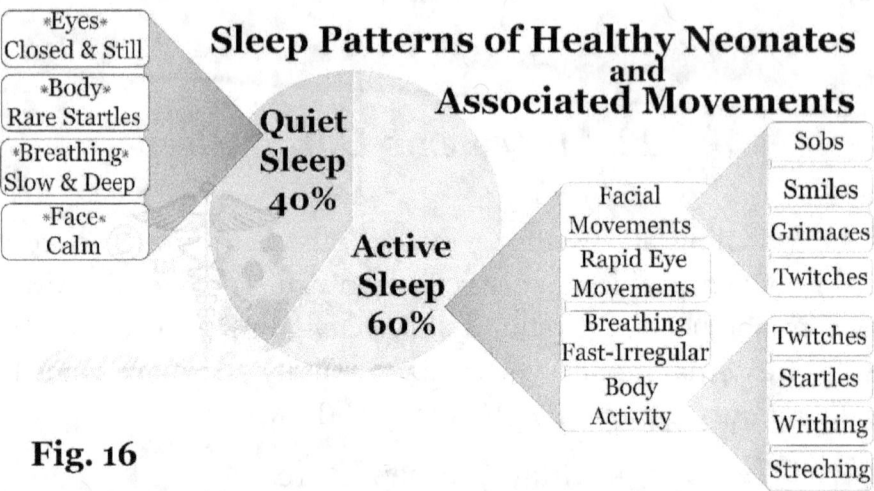

Fig. 16

Though an occasional startle or twitch may be spotted during deep sleep, most movements that arouse concern are seen during active sleep (Fig. 16). Signals from the Pons at the base of the brain initiate active sleep. These nerve impulses travel through Thalamus and spread over to Cerebral Cortex, the seat of perception, learning, and enacting. The cortex tries to make meaning out of the random clues transmitted from the pons during active sleep. It creates dreams, bizarre images, and illogical experiences, out of the fragmented activity of the brain and tries to act on them. Moreover, the pons also sends impulses that shut off neurons in the spinal cord, and prevent peripheral muscles from moving in sleep.

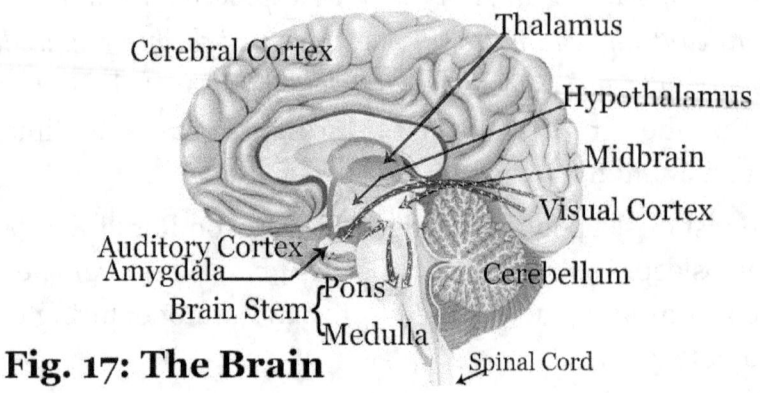

Fig. 17: The Brain

During infancy, the complex network of nerves is yet evolving. The two main *axonal pathways involved in the initiation of movements are the corticospinal tract (Fig.7), and the **corticobulbar tract. The immature corticospinal tract is unable to bring about an efficient inhibitory control on the motor-system***. This is probably why young infants are prone to sudden outbursts of a

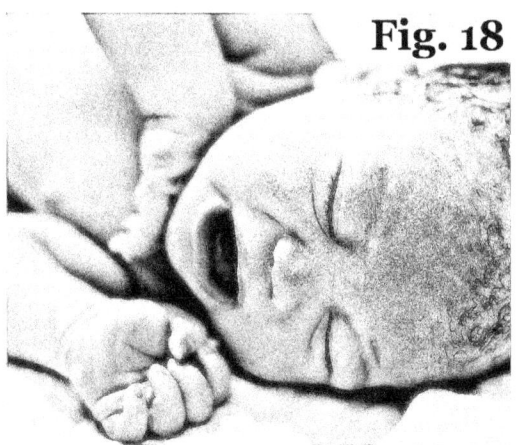

Fig. 18

Baby reacting to bizarre images in sleep, created by the fragmented activity of the brain.

variety of movements and gestures during their active sleep phase, and at times even when they are awake. But the literature to support this is grossly inadequate.

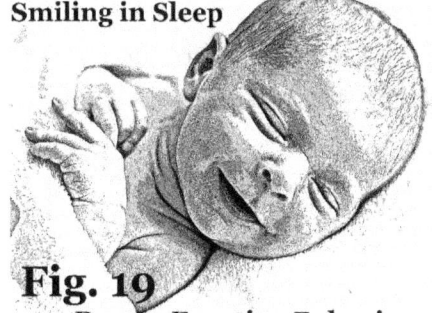

Smiling in Sleep

Fig. 19

Dream Enacting Behaviour

Nevertheless, Dream Enacting Behaviours have been extensively studied in older children and adults, in whom it could be associated with an underlying neurological deficit. But *in infants, enacting during active sleep is believed to be the normal stimulation for healthy development of the brain.*

During early infancy critical and quick maturational changes in the brain have been documented and supported by EEG pattern changes, which reflect the dynamic character of the nervous system development.

----

*Axon: Long thread-like part of a nerve cell, which carries impulses from the cell body to other cells (Fig.14)

**Corticobulbar Tract: Nerve bundles that connect the motor cortex to the pyramids (Fig. 7) in the Medulla (Fig. 17)

***Motor System: The part of the central nervous system involved in effectuating coordinated purposeful movements.

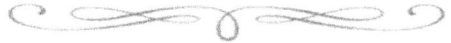

13. Rhythmic Movement Disorder

Purposeless rhythmic movements of one or the other part of the body during sleep and sleepiness are seen in almost 50% of babies under 3 months of age. Many well cared for normal older infants bang or roll their head while falling asleep, more so if they are left alone in their cribs or playpen. This causes considerable concern in young parents. Not only do they worry about the injury such meaningless movements may inflict, but also for the possibility of an underlying neurological defect.

A normal phenomenon

Intense rhythmic motor activity (RMA) at sleep time, which is not associated with altered clarity of mind, is a transient voluntary phenomenon in healthy and developmentally normal infants.

Stress buster

Most babies, between 6 and 36 months, indulge in variety of rhythmic movements, sometimes for the sheer pleasure of activity, and at other times to overcome stress. It is their way to cope with restraints that hinders their freedom of action. Inadequate playful interaction, bodily pain, and obstacles stir up anxiety, helplessness, and frustration in them.

An unusual variety of childhood parasomnia*

The repetitive motor events occur in several different forms. They can involve any part of the body; head, trunk, or extremities. Body rocking, head banging and head rolling are the most common. Leg and hand banging are also frequently encountered.

The duration of rhythmic activity varies, but seldom exceed for more than 15 min. It typically occurs during the transition from wakefulness to sleep, and may recur at intervals that differ from child to child. In some cases, rhythmic movements may continue throughout the night, at about 2 hours intervals within the 24 hours of sleep-wake cycle.

Attributed to normal nervous system development

Sleep-related rhythmic movements are common among normal children. They are typically seen during the changeover from the state of sleep to wakefulness. Hence the name is "sleep-wake transition disorder". Its onset is in early infancy, and spontaneous resolution is usual. Most kids get over sleep-related rhythmic movements by 36 months of age. It is noteworthy that the span of sleep-wake transition disorder coincides with the major developmental phase of motor skills and posture control, both of which are essential for performing day to day activities effectively.

The significance of the sleep-wake cycle

Infant's sleep-wake cycle involves transitions between four different states: wakefulness, drowsiness, rapid eye movement (REM) sleep, which is associated with dreaming, and quiet sleep (Non-REM sleep: Fig. 15). The neurological "barriers" that separate these states are functionally immature during initial months of life. So is the thalamo-cortical reticular system (Fig. 20), which inhibits voluntary muscular activities, and brings about generalized limpness of the body that is commonly associated with sleep. This physiological immaturity of the inhibitory thalamo-cortical reticular system is believed to be the cause of sleep related rhythmic movements in infancy and toddlerhood.

Pathological loss of inhibitory cortex function

Rhythmic movements that are clearly derived from a dysfunction of motor control during sleep, and constitute true sleep-related motor disorders also exist. Therefore, the normal physiological phenomenon, which most kids spontaneously grow out of, need to be differentiated from a symptom of some concomitant neurological disorders.

In its benign form it affects infants and toddlers in a transient and self-limited fashion. But *when it persists beyond 3 years of age, it is often a sign of poor mental development.*

Pathological rhythmic movements persist for a much longer period. They may relapse or develop anew later in childhood. In some cases, relationships between rhythmic movement disorder and epilepsy have also been found. In these cases a detailed neurological evaluation is indicated. EEG and Polysomnography** may help in the diagnosis.

Treatment

1. Medical evaluation is a must:
   Rhythmic movement disorder is essentially benign behaviour that heralds no treatment. Nevertheless, medical evaluation is a must to differentiate severe episodes of purposeless stereotyped movements during sleep from the nocturnal seizure disorder.

2. Pad the sides of the crib:
   There is always the fear of injury with vigorous head banging. Padding the sides of the crib not only prevents trauma to the infant but also minimizes the noise, which could be disturbing, particularly at nights.

3. Train banging the head without letting it touch the pillow:
   For children in whom rhythmic movements persist into sleep, a unique therapy has been suggested, in which the child is made to practice head banging without actually letting the head touch the pillow. Over time child learns to stop short of the pillow even in sleep. This prevents injury.

4. Restraining a child in hope of stopping the movements is not advisable.

5. Watch over:
   Many times the cause for child's unease is negligence, deprivation, or child abuse, and the head banging is the baby's way to express her distress. Infants and toddlers need safe and nurturing environment for healthy development. Optimal care and interaction satisfy their social and emotional needs.

6. Medication is not necessary in most cases:
   Only a few with a severe form of sleep related rhythmic movement disorder may benefit from medicines.

----

*Parasomnia: It is a group of unusual behaviour of the nervous system during sleep, which usually occurs due to partial arousals during the transitions between wakefulness and non-REM sleep, or wakefulness and REM sleep. It may comprise of any combination of activities or behaviours along with emotions and perceptions, while falling asleep, during sleep, between different stages of sleep, or during arousal from sleep. Dreams, sleep walking, sleep related eating disorder, enuresis, sleep paralysis, sleep sex and sleep aggression are also different types of parasomnia.

**Polysomnography: It is an overnight study of the pattern of sleep on those who suffer from sleep disorder. It records the brain waves, oxygen level in the blood, heart rate, breathing pattern, eye movements, and all forms of muscle activity during sleep. The word is derived from the Greek, "poly," means many, "somno," means sleep, and "graphy" means to record - often in an image form.

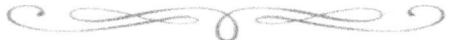

14. Myoclonus in Babies

Sudden rhythmic jerks in a newly born baby send the parents into jitters. They fear fits, a well-known manifestation of nervous system disorder. They rush to their doctor for help. Grandma gives a cursory glance at the infant's moving fingers, and comments in a carefree manner, "ah, she is counting money in her dream".

Dream?

Yes, "dreams and not fits" is probably more near the truth! Brief irregular bursts of involuntary movements do occur in normal newborns. Though predominantly seen during sleep, they are not due to dreams of present or past life. They are benign neonatal sleep myoclonus.

What is myoclonus?

Myoclonus is an involuntary burst of irregular muscular activity that produces movements that are neither symmetric nor synchronous. The visible jerking movements are termed positive myoclonus, whereas sudden limpness due to uncontrolled muscle relaxation is called negative myoclonus.

Myoclonic jerks come unexpectedly in a baby who is fast asleep, and they last only for a few seconds. Though each episode is brief, many episodes occur in a day. Further, myoclonic bursts often come in a sequence, and continue for several minutes. They are of a much higher magnitude than tremulousness in normal newborns. Therefore, they are commonly mistaken for seizures, but like jitteriness, they too are the outcome of a yet developing nervous system.

Benign sleep myoclonus in newborns

This innocent self-limiting movement disorder was first described in 1982. The precise cause of this condition is yet unknown, and till date the available literature is limited.

It is characterized by positive myoclonus that occurs exclusively during sleep. It is commonly seen in healthy full-term and near-term newborns, but only a few, who fear neonatal seizures, seek medical help. Consequently, the present reports show a maximum incidence of 3.0 cases per 1000 births.

It presents within 2 weeks of birth, and 95% of the cases resolve on their own by 3-6 months of age. Some of the remaining 5% continue having episodic jerks beyond the second year of life. These infants are born healthy, and they continue to be healthy in spite of the persistent seizure like muscular activity.

No neurological defect is noted; neither clinically nor on EEG (electroencephalogram) taken during or after the episodes. Laboratory evaluation also does not show any electrolyte or metabolic derangement. Babies sleep undisturbed through the myoclonic march, which ends abruptly when they wake up.

To be precise, neonatal sleep myoclonus leaves no sequelae. It neither endangers the development nor the learning abilities of the children affected, and it does not increase the risk of convulsive disorders in them.

Presentation of sleep myoclonus varies widely

Myoclonic jerks in neonates are seen mainly during quiet sleep (Fig. 16). But they can also occur in active sleep, when they are often mistaken for active sleep related twitches and startles.

The brief shock like jerky movements come in symmetric or asymmetric clusters, each of which can last up to 30 minutes. They are repetitive, and typically bilateral, but can also be unilateral, focal, multifocal, generalized or marching. The muscle contractions can involve one or more limbs at a time, which produce movements that are neither uniform nor do they recur together at regular intervals. The duration of each episode is variable too. Consequently, the prolonged episodes are often mistaken for status epilepticus (Fifth day fits, pg. 106).

The upper limbs are more frequently affected than the lower, and the small muscles of the fingers and toes more than the large proximal ones. Rarely trunk muscles may also show myoclonic jerks, which may be isolated or repetitive, but the face muscles are never involved during the neonatal period. All the jerking is typically during sleep. *If the abnormal movements are noticed seen when the baby is awake, a diagnosis other than benign sleep myoclonus should be considered.*

Proposed neurophysiological mechanisms

Primarily benign myoclonus in newborns is believed to be a type of sleep disorder, which results from inappropriate activation of the physiological systems. This concept is further supported by the fact that the jerky movements are seen in the period when infants' sleep pattern is maturing. Therefore, it has been linked to maturation of reticular activating system and their serotonergic pathways*, which normally suppress motor response (movements) during sleep. The transient imbalance of the important inhibitory neurotransmitters during this phase of development, could be the cause of disturbed reticular activating system functions.

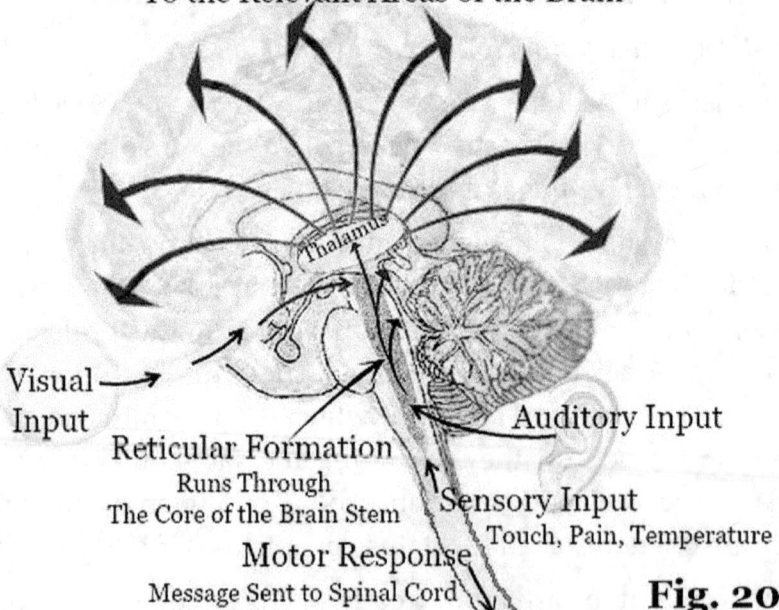

Reticular Activating System
Regulates Wakefulness & Sleep-Wake Transitions
Filters the Inputs and Passes Important Information
To the Relevant Areas of the Brain

Thalamus

Visual Input

Auditory Input

Reticular Formation
Runs Through
The Core of the Brain Stem

Sensory Input
Touch, Pain, Temperature

Motor Response
Message Sent to Spinal Cord

Fig. 20

Another cause for the myoclonus in neonates could be the sudden withdrawal of opiate-like drugs. Opioid receptors are widely distributed in the brain and the spinal cord. They are activated only when endorphins and other neuro-active molecules with opioid-like structures, produced within the nerve cells, bind to them. The impulse thus generated has an inhibitory effect on the target neurons. It lowers its excitability and reduces the release of neurotransmitters. *Loss of this inhibitory control explains the cause of many fold higher incidence of sleep myoclonus in infants of mothers who take opiate containing drugs during pregnancy.*

Nevertheless, the myoclonic activity can originate from any part of the nervous system (cortex, brainstem, spinal cord or nerve), and at times as a reflex phenomenon in response to sensory stimuli, like repetitive sounds, rocking, and movements during automobile rides.

A few studies have indicated that some of these cases could have a familial predisposition. A genetic link to parasomnia** and migraine has also been suggested. The mode of transmission is not yet clear. Boys and girls are equally affected.

Avoid medications

Benign neonatal sleep myoclonus is a self-limiting disorder. Even though myoclonic episodes closely resemble seizures, no medications are indicated for its treatment. Use of anti-epileptic drugs; benzodiazepines and chlorpromazine, prolong and worsen the involuntary jerky movements in these infants, which resolve when the medication is stopped. In contrast, early therapy is essential for neonatal seizures, which may be the first and the only sign of an underlying treatable neurological disorder. *The diagnosis and treatment should, therefore, be decided only after good medical evaluation.*

A diagnosis of exclusion

Benign neonatal sleep myoclonus is a diagnosis of exclusion. *Differentiation between epileptic and non-epileptic myoclonus is critical for appropriate management. It is therefore vital to seek a professional opinion in all such cases.* Video recording of the paroxysmal movements could help in the diagnosis.

The classical clinical presentation and normal EEG, along with the relatively normal behaviour of the baby is the key to the diagnosis. In addition, the jerks of sleep myoclonus are uniquely worsened when restrained. The epileptic myoclonus, on the other hand, is neither triggered by stimuli nor suppressed or modified by restraining the affected body part.

Other causes of myoclonus in neonatal period

Symptomatic myoclonus

1. Hypoxic–ischemic brain injury
   Poor oxygen and blood supply to the brain

2. Severe intraventricular haemorrhage
   Brain haemorrhage

3. Glycine encephalopathy**
   Inborn shortage of an enzyme that normally breaks down glycine; a building block of proteins and a chemical messenger that transmits signals in the brain.

4. Drug withdrawal symptom
   a.   After intravenous benzodiazepines therapy
   b.   Babies of opioid dependent mothers

Epileptic myoclonus

1. Epileptic myoclonic encephalopathy

2. Early infantile epileptic encephalopathy

----

*Serotonergic Pathways: The nerve endings that release and are stimulated by serotonin, a neuroactive chemical. These nerves are found in many areas of the brain. They regulate the body clock, pain tolerance, appetite and satiety controls, learning, emotional processing, behaviour, mood and much more.

** Encephalopathy: A disease in which the functioning of the brain is affected by some agent or condition such as viral infection or toxins in the blood.

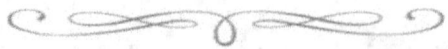

15. Benign Myoclonus of Early Infancy

Benign myoclonus of early infancy (BMEI) is a rare movement disorder wherein neurologically healthy infants present with a spectrum of abnormal movements. Generally, the onset is between three and nine months of age. A few have late onset, but later than 15 months of age has not yet been documented. The abnormal muscular activity disappears spontaneously, latest by 30 months of age. It does not normally leave behind any ill effects on child's development. Till date, the underlying cause for this disorder is not known, nor are provoking factors determined.

Various abnormal movements seen in BMEI include myoclonic jerks, muscle spasms, brief tonic contractions, shuddering, and nonepileptic limpness (negative myoclonus - pg. 62). These differences may, however, be quite subtle. Moreover, about 9% of the cases manifest a combination of the different type of abnormal muscular activity.

Typically, the attacks are sudden and brief shuddering of the trunk and the head, without changes in the level of alertness and responsiveness. Less frequently, there may be stiffening of the limbs, head drops or loss of tone in the trunk. Each episode usually lasts only for a second or two, which, in most cases, come in clusters and many times a day, but not necessarily every day. The intensity of each episode varies from inconspicuous movements to vigorous jerking of the limbs. These fits like movements do not involve any particular group of muscles. Nor do they have lateralizing features that would indicate the area of the brain from which the abnormal impulses could be originating.

The variability of presentation, though not quite conspicuous, confuses this "innocent self-limiting involuntary movement disorder" with several non-epileptic and epileptic fits of early infancy. The commonest being the harmless "sleep myoclonus" on one hand, and a devastating infantile spasms epilepsy, the West syndrome, on the other.

Distinguishing features

In contrast to benign neonatal sleep myoclonus, BMEI is hardly ever seen in the neonatal period. The myoclonic episodes in this disorder occur when the infant is awake, and seldom in sleep. Apart from that, this rare condition is very similar to sleep myoclonus (pg. 62).

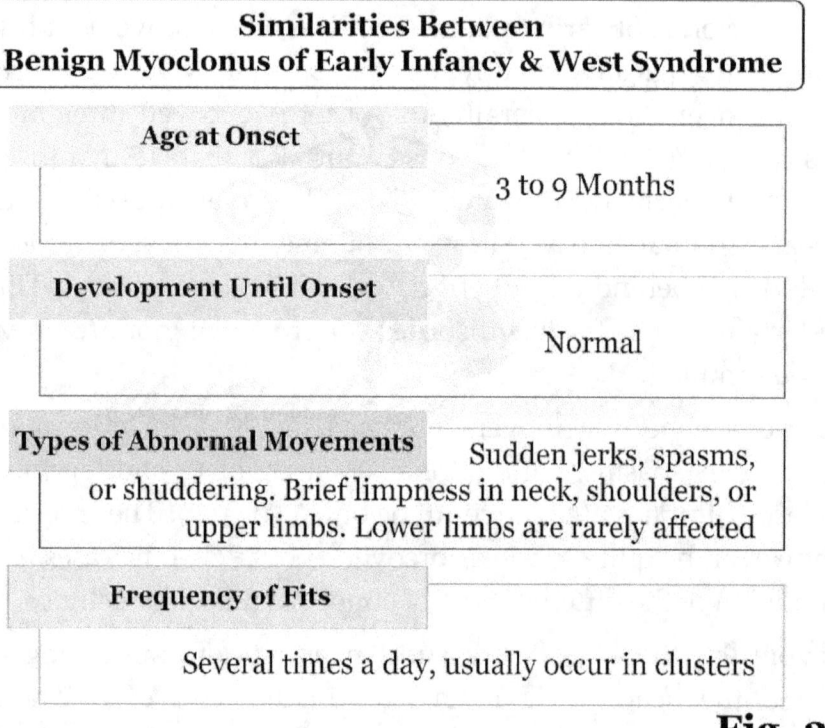

Similarities Between Benign Myoclonus of Early Infancy & West Syndrome

Age at Onset	3 to 9 Months
Development Until Onset	Normal
Types of Abnormal Movements	Sudden jerks, spasms, or shuddering. Brief limpness in neck, shoulders, or upper limbs. Lower limbs are rarely affected
Frequency of Fits	Several times a day, usually occur in clusters

Fig. 21

It is also clearly different from the West syndrome:

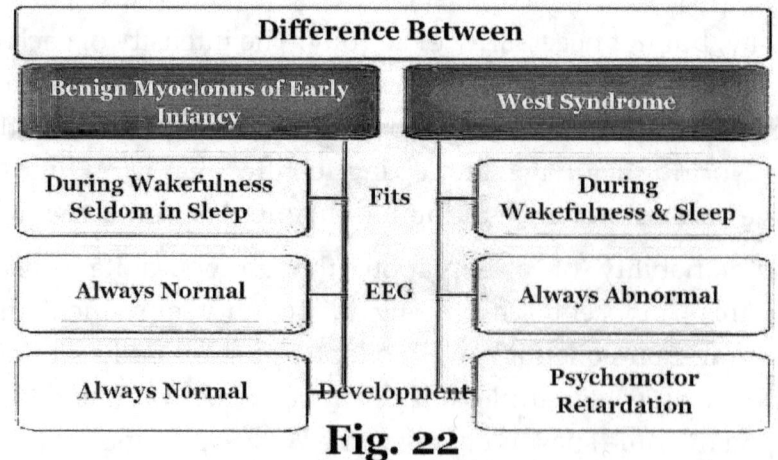

Difference Between

Benign Myoclonus of Early Infancy		West Syndrome
During Wakefulness Seldom in Sleep	Fits	During Wakefulness & Sleep
Always Normal	EEG	Always Abnormal
Always Normal	Development	Psychomotor Retardation

Fig. 22

In cases of BMEI, involuntary shudders and tonic spasms can easily be mistaken for "infantile spasms", an epilepsy syndrome.

The attacks, in both these disorders, are commonly associated with feeding. Its age of onset further adds to the confusion. But the two hallmark of "infantile spasms epilepsy", developmental regression and chaotic brain waves on EEG (hypsarrhythmia) are never seen in cases of "benign myoclonus of early infancy". EEG evaluation of babies suffering from of BMEI is consistently normal; even during the episodes. Video-EEG monitoring, therefore, helps to clinch the diagnosis.

As opposed to the West syndrome, BMEI has a self-limited course. The frequency of fits decreases within 3 months of onset. Complete spontaneous resolution occurs before 2 years of age in the majority. It does not jeopardize the development of the skills, language, or intellect of the child. Nevertheless, 1 in 6 of the affected children tends to be hyperactive, but they do not suffer from the related learning disabilities.

Antiepileptic medications are not recommended for control of this innocent involuntary movement disorder. But if given due to a diagnostic dilemma, they do not alter the course. Affected babies suffer no ill effects, nor is their risk of developing true epilepsy increased. They grow to be healthy babies.

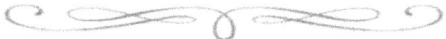

16. Sleep Starts

It is common to find an infant wake up with a startle just after having been put to sleep. The whole event resembles the startle reflex in response to a sudden loss of support. Similarly, during sleep starts babies feel as if they are falling.

Sleep Starts

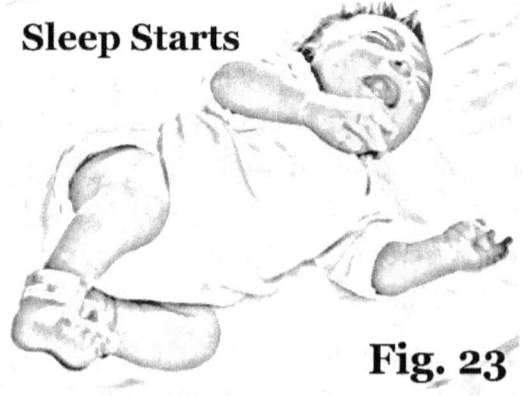

Fig. 23

They go into sudden contractions of one or more body parts, usually involving the trunk and all extremities simultaneously, and let out a cry of fear. The mother enfolds the baby in her arms in a reassuring fashion, and then the baby usually sleeps through. Some babies may experience 3-4 jolts before they actually go into deep sleep, which parents associate with infant's ability to sense that the mother has moved away.

Normal variant of sleep related movement disorder

Sleep starts, also known as hypnic* jerks, are a common form of myoclonus. In this the child experiences a sudden uncontrollable "jolt", usually of the whole body, which occurs just before the child gets into the deep sleep phase of non REM sleep (Fig. 15).

Hypnic jerks are brief. They usually last for less than a second. Like benign sleep myoclonus (pg. 62), they are the harmless effect of the normal transition from wake to sleep. However, the EEG taken during the episode shows alpha-waves** immediately after the jerk. Such an EEG can easily be mistaken for epileptic myoclonic seizures especially in infants and toddlers.

Common occurrence

Sleep starts are seen in all age groups, and equally in both sexes. 2-3 consecutive jolts in babies under 6 months of age are commonly ignored as normal startle reflex of infancy. And with the advancement of age, the frequency of sleep starts falls so low, that most parents don't even consider taking a medical opinion. When they do, it being the commonest sleep related movement disorder in children, the doctors often dismiss them as usual phenomena encountered during the course of normal childhood development. More so, because the crop of hypnic jerks does not leave behind any ill effect on children's health, development or intellect. Yet, the documented overall prevalence of sleep starts is 70%, of which only 1 in 10 report daily symptoms.

A quasi physiological*** motor phenomenon

The search for the precise cause of sleep starts continues. Most of the studies are done on adults, and it is generally agreed that they are an essential part of the sleep onset process. They are believed to arise from sudden descending nerve impulses that originate in reticular formation (Fig. 20) and escape down the system due to a brief imbalance of important inhibitory neurotransmitters during the wake and sleep transition phase. This causes a brief body jolt that usually lasts for less than a second. Along with it occurs activation of the autonomic nervous system****, which is marked by rapid breathing and increase in the heart rate.

Babies are not vocal, but if they were, like most adult patients, they too would have reported sleep starts associated subjective feelings, such as tingling or floating sensation, visualization of flashes of light or a dream, hearing noises, etc. These sensory experiences can occur without the physical jolt.

High intake of chocolates and caffeine containing drinks by nursing mothers, exposure to secondhand tobacco smoke, an erratic lifestyle of parents and a hereditary predisposition are some common causes of frequent episodes of hypnic jerks and associated sensory perceptions. Actual disturbances during sleep, like sound or skin contact, can also evoke cluster of sensory or motor sleep starts.

Sleep starts may reflect neurological abnormality

Regardless of the fact that brief cluster of sleep starts can occur in normal infants, all forms of repetitive sensory and motor activity during sleep should be recognized and clearly differentiated from epileptic seizures.

Intense and/or repetitive sleep starts in infancy could be the manifestation of hypoxic***** brain injury in the womb, at birth or thereafter. In other cases, they may represent infantile spasms, epilepsy, hyperekplexia****** or other genetic predisposed neurological abnormalities.

In neurologically impaired children, the normal swing between sleep and wakefulness is enhanced during the drowsy state. This is because of the failure of physiological inhibitory influence of the compromised pyramidal tracts*******. Therefore, in such cases sleep starts often acquire the tendency to recur at intervals. Usually, these infants have a correlating medical history and neurological findings. Their clinical presentation frequently resembles epileptic attack, and the available EEG findings are scanty. Both these together make diagnosis difficult, more so in infants and toddlers, in whom the incidence of non-rapid eye movement sleep disorders is the highest.

What should the parents do?

Parents need not get unduly frightened. It is important to note that the majority of reported jerks at the onset of sleep are common sleep starts. But it is also important to be aware that, when they spot intense purposeless movements in their child a detailed neurological evaluation is a must.

Hypnic*: The word comes from Greek word Hypnos which means sleep.

Alpha waves:** They are a type of brain waves recorded on electroencephalography (EEG). They predominantly originate from the occipital lobe during wakeful relaxation with closed eyes, and are reduced on opening the eyes, with drowsiness and sleep.

Physiological***: Relating to normal functions of the body.

Autonomic Nervous System****: The part of the nervous system that controls vital functions of body organs, which cannot be voluntarily altered. For example, breathing, heart beats, digestive processes and so on.

Hypoxic*****: Low oxygen supply to the tissue

Hyperekplexia******: It is an abnormal startle response to sudden, potentially threatening stimuli of any type, particularly a loud sound. The stimulus induces a protective reaction, which is often widespread and violent. The reaction comprises of sudden contractions of the head, neck, spinal, and sometimes, limb musculature, which may end in an involuntary shout, jolt, jump, or fall. The exaggerated reaction to stimuli is probably due to inherited deficiency of inhibitory neurotransmitters; glycine or GABA. Both autosomal dominant and recessive inheritance are known. The responsible gene is localized on chromosome 5q.

The Pyramidal Tracts******* (Fig. 7): They are bundle of nerve fibres that originate in the brain (cerebral cortex) and travel down, some to the brainstem (Fig. 36), and the rest to different levels of the spinal cord, known as corticospinal tracts. Together they control the body movements.

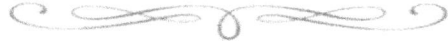

Section III
Rare Causes

17. Pyridoxine Dependent Seizures

Pyridoxine is the generic name for vitamin B6. In its active form (pyridoxal 5'-phosphate), it serves as a coenzyme to convert food into fuel, helps make antibodies*, and contributes to the production of hemoglobin. It plays a crucial role in the synthesis of neurotransmitters (pg.46) such as serotonin, dopamine, epinephrine, norepinephrine, and gamma-aminobutyric acid (GABA).

Pyridoxine dependency is a rare cause of fits in newborns

Till date only a few cases have been diagnosed, and so the literature available is also sparse. The reason for including it in this book is that it is fully curable. Parents' awareness of this entity should help in early diagnosis, and thereby prompt treatment of this distressing disorder. The onset of the disease is often in the womb. Some mothers have been able to identify excessive abnormal movements in their unborn baby.

Mode of Inheritance of Pyridoxine Dependent Seizures
Autosomal Recessive

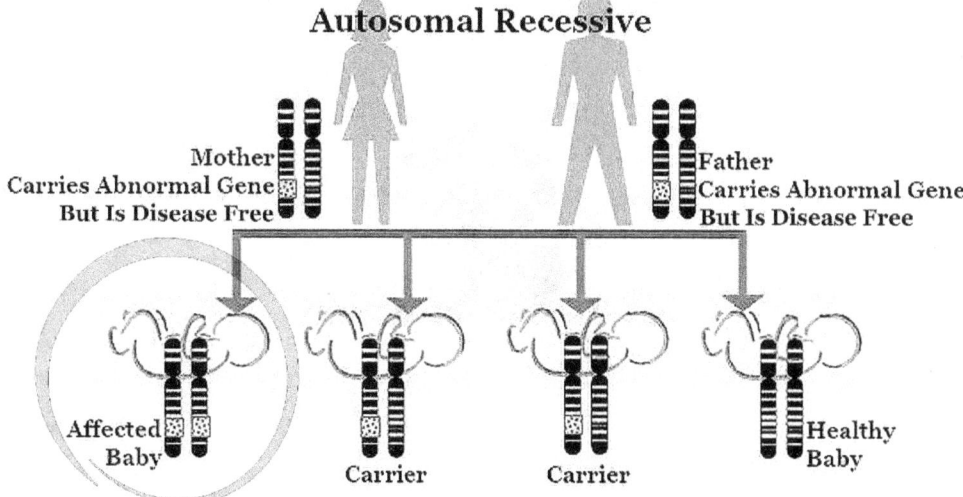

Mother
Carries Abnormal Gene
But Is Disease Free

Father
Carries Abnormal Gene
But Is Disease Free

Affected Baby

Carrier

Carrier

Healthy Baby

Note: Only 1 in 4 Chances To Inherit The Abnormal Gene From Both The Parents

Fig. 24

It is not the dietary deficiency of the vitamin that causes seizures, but an inborn abnormality in the pyridoxine-dependent synthesis of the inhibitory neurotransmitter (GABA). The defect is usually inherited by autosomal recessive mode (Fig. 24), though a few new mutations** are also documented.

Fits

Pyridoxine-dependent epilepsy presents with different types of fits; generalized or partial seizures, episodes of limpness, infantile spasms and myoclonic jerks. Typically, within the first few days of birth, the affected baby presents with prolonged seizures, which are almost impossible to control, even on administration of anticonvulsant drugs. Episodes of status epilepticus are thus common.

The diagnosis

Though Pipecolic acid in plasma and cerebrospinal fluid is considered a possible metabolic marker for this disorder, the quick response to pyridoxine supplementation clinches the diagnosis. The EEG in these cases is also uniquely abnormal. The pattern of generalized burst-suppression activity in neonates is believed to be highly suggestive of the diagnosis. Brain imaging (CT and MRI) may show a variety of abnormalities. Finally, the genetic testing would reveal the abnormal gene.

Timely treatment can prevent developmental disabilities

All seizures of pyridoxine-dependent epilepsy stop within minutes of pyridoxine supplementation, and the EEG normalize during the next few hours. On the other hand, delay in treatment results in developmental disabilities. Intravenous vitamin B6 is therefore given as a therapeutic trial to establish the diagnosis.

Despite being a vitamin, the dose in which it would be effective is not devoid of danger. Precautions need to be taken against the possible collapse of vital functions. Intravenous administration of vitamin B6 is done under continuous EEG monitoring. Necessary baseline blood evaluation is also done before giving the B6 shot.

----

*Antibody: Protein of body's primary defense system. They combine with substances which the body recognizes as alien, such as bacteria, viruses and other foreign substances, and induce their inactivation.

** **Mutation:** It creates slightly different versions of the same genes. The resultant variant form can be transmitted to subsequent generations, like any other gene. It is the ultimate way to evolution. It explains the variations seen in human race; colour, height, body build, behaviour pattern, and susceptibility to disease. A few mutations are however harmful and lead to diseases.

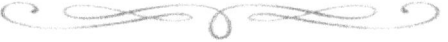

18. Inborn Tremulous Movement of The Chin

An involuntary, intermittent shaking of the chin that is first noticed during the initial hours after birth, which at times persists through infancy, toddler years, childhood and beyond. This is the "hereditary chin trembling", a rare genetic disorder, which is also known as "hereditary chin myoclonus".

The defective gene is usually passed down from the parent who as a child suffered similar chin tremors, though their intensity and duration would have decreased with age. In some, it could be the result of a new autosomal dominant gene mutation, wherein the baby is the first to be affected in the family. Nevertheless, the children of this baby

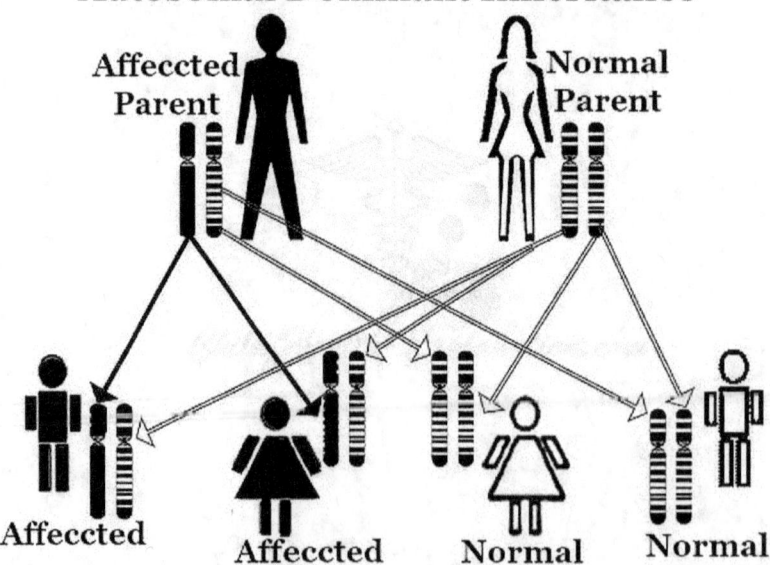

Autosomal Dominant Inheritance

Affeccted Parent

Normal Parent

Affeccted

Affeccted

Normal

Normal

*Irrespective of the sex of the affected parent,
each of their offspring (also irrespective of the sex) has
50-50 chances of being affected.*

Fig. 25

would be at risk of acquiring the movement disorder by the pattern of autosomal dominant inheritance.

Despite the fact that boys and girls are equally at risk of inheriting an autosomal dominant disease, the incidence of chin trembling (Geniospasm) is found to be a little more in the male infants. The affected babies are remarkably healthy except for the intermittent tremulous activity of the chin (mentalis muscle). They neither have any neurological impairment nor any other abnormal movement. Their intelligence and skills development is normal.

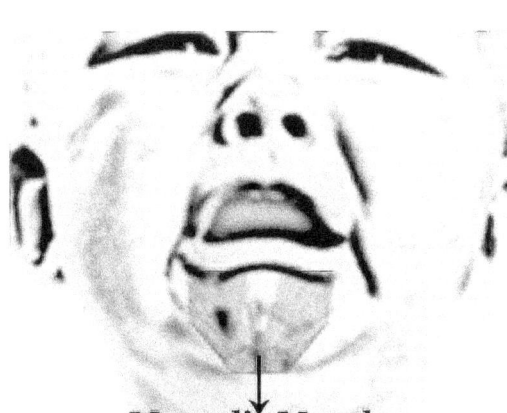

Mentalis Muscle

*A paired central muscle of the lower lip.
Situated at the tip of the chin.
It elevates and wrinkles skin of chin, and
protrudes lower lip.*

Fig. 26

In short, fit like recurrent rhythmic trembling of the chin, which typically becomes apparent in infancy or in early childhood, is believed to be a harmless movement disorder.

Social impairment

The tremulous chin can, however, be a serious cause of social uneasiness and peer ridicule at a very tender age. The recurrent bouts of involuntary up and down movements of lower lip and chin impede speech. Inaccurate articulation distorts communication and hinders reading and recitation. The social embarrassment that results, prevents the child to participate freely in school activities. Socially isolated friendless children become common targets for peer victimization.

The patient has no control over the trembling chin

In most infants, the chin tremors occur spontaneously. But in some, they are noted to be triggered by stress, concentration, and emotions. Each episode may last from a few seconds to several minutes. In a few severe cases, the tremors may even spread to the upper lip.

Treatment and prognosis

The frequency and intensity of these attacks tend to reduce as the age advances. Usually, no treatment is required, and when it was tried it was of little benefit if any.

Is hereditary chin trembling a variant of essential tremor?

No.

Unlike chin trembling of infancy, essential tremor (pg. 83) is a slowly progressive disorder that rarely begins in infancy.

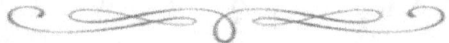

19. Essential Tremor

"Essential tremor" (ET) is hardly ever diagnosed in children, though it is the most common movement disorder among the adults, many of whom report its onset in childhood. It is probably because it develops gradually and subtly. As a result, the tremors in children are not severe enough to interfere with their day to day activities.

The prevalence

On the basis of spirals drawn by school children ranging from 6 to 16 years of age, a recent study determined that a little over 2% of them suffered from mild to moderate tremors, but only a few sought medical advice. The number of cases recorded in pediatric age group thus falls to only about 20% of all types of childhood movement disorders.

The awareness will probably help overcome the bias of "essential tremor" being a disease of the adults, and help early recognition of the disorder in children, some of whom suffer from the tender age of 2, or even less.

Predisposing Factors

Essential tremor is an important autosomal dominant disorder (Fig. 25), which is usually inherited but may also be the outcome of a new mutation. The severity of the disorder varies from family to family. It was first described in the nineteenth century. At that time no apparent external cause could be ascertained for this slowly and insidiously worsening movement disorder, hence the prefix "essential" came into being.

Characteristics

The commonest and probably the only, presenting symptom of the disorder is tremulousness, which most frequently is symmetrical, and is typically seen in both hands and arms when they are being used or held against gravity. Nevertheless, some cases present only with the tremors of the head. But tremors of any other part of the body would be consistent with the diagnosis of ET only if they coexist with the tremors of arms and hands, or head.

The involuntary rhythmic shaking of the hands, at about six to 10 times in a second, is best noted when the child is eating with a spoon, lifting an object like a cup of milk, or writing. ET can also affect the voice in a few, but probably not that of young children. Tremors of the legs, though rare, indicates juvenile Parkinson Disease.

Any associated nervous system dysfunction negates the diagnosis of essential tremor, so also the history of exposure to neurotoxins. Neuroimaging studies are normal in this condition. Nevertheless, the factors that disturb the mental balance do exaggerate tremulousness, like in stress, anxiety, lack of sleep, or tobacco and coffee intake.

Diagnosis of essential tremor can be confusing

Till date, it is seldom diagnosed in children below the age of 5 years. However, the parents often retrospectively recall tremulousness from the early months of the child's life.

It is popularly accepted as a single symptom disease, but the possibility of associated dystonia, myoclonus, and impairment of the movements of the face muscles cannot be totally ruled out, especially in affected infants and toddlers.

Moreover, the shuddering attacks in infancy are believed to be the forerunner of essential tremor disorder and/or dystonia in later life. On the other hand, innocent tremors of infancy can be mistaken for early onset of essential tremor disorder.

A good neurological evaluation by an expert is, therefore, a must for an early and appropriate management of these cases, particularly in children whose blood relative is known to be suffering from dystonia or Parkinsonism.

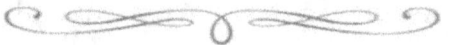

20. Head Tilt: Torticollis of Infancy

Torticollis* is a type of movement disorder wherein the neck muscles that control the position of the head go into unwanted activity. As a result, the neck twists such that the head leans abnormally towards one of the shoulders. "Abnormally" here means that it is not necessarily in accord with the gaze alignment.

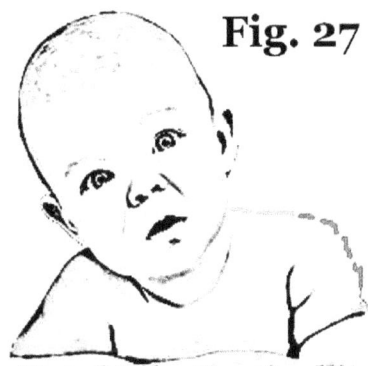

Fig. 27

Head Tilt: Torticollis

During the first few weeks, torticollis should be suspected if parents notice that their baby always turns the same side of her face toward the mattress. Over time, this can cause flattening of head on the side of the tilt. Consequently, the face may appear asymmetrical. The infants in whom the treatment is delayed, develop permanent facial deformity, and the movements of their head get restricted.

Common causes of abnormal head tilt

Fig. 28

Sternocleidomastoid Muscle Lump

1. Lump in sternocleidomastoid, a major muscle of the neck, which joins the base of the skull to the collarbone, is the commonest form of Torticollis seen in neonatal practice.

2. Postural

3. Abnormal position in womb.

4. Congenital absence or shortening of sternomastoid muscle.

5. Acute atlantoaxial subluxation (partial dislocation of the first two vertebrae of the neck)

6. Hemivertebrae, an inborn wedge shaped deformity of one or more small neck bones, which causes the spine to twist.

Fig:29

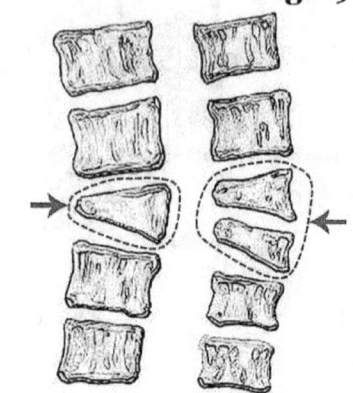

7. Tumor in posterior fossa of the skull.

8. Spasmodic with Sandifer syndrome (pg. 90)

9. Pyogenic cervical (neck spine) spondylitis - Bacterial infection of soft disc of cartilage in between 2 vertebrae

10. Neck abscess

11. Inflammation of the lymph nodes of the neck.

Hemivertebrae

Fig. 30

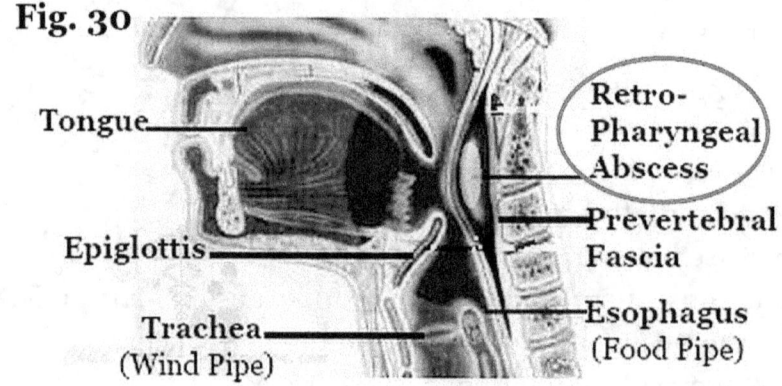

12. Retropharyngeal abscess is collection of pus at the back of the throat in small space between the food pipe and the prevertebral fascia. Usually seen in toddler years, but can occur at any age.

13. Benign paroxysmal torticollis of infancy (BPTI)

All of the above are rare, and their outcome varies depending on the underlying cause. Accept for spasmodic torticollis associated with Sandifer syndrome (pg. 90) and Benign Paroxysmal Torticollis of Infancy (pg. 87), none others come as fits and starts.

----

*Torticollis: The medical term for the sideward tilt of the head, while the backward head tilt is called retrocollis.

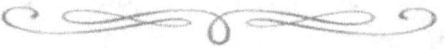

21. Benign Paroxysmal Torticollis of Infancy

Benign paroxysmal torticollis of infancy (BPTI) is an innocent self-limited functional disorder. It is characterized by a needless head tilt in healthy babies that recurs every few weeks. First described almost half a century ago, in 1969 by the neurologist Snyder, its awareness is yet found wanting among children's health care providers.

Incidence

Girls are more frequently affected; girls to boys ratio being 3:1, but the exact prevalence of BPTI remains unknown. The cases of periodic head tilt in infancy seldom draw medical attention; partly because the disorder causes no discomfort to the baby. A few cases that are diagnosed also fall off records as the symptoms resolve completely before the child starts the schooling.

Onset

The onset of this episodic functional disorder can be anytime after birth. Most cases present in first 12 weeks of life, but late onset (until 2½ years of age) has also been noted. Initially, the infant may present only with abnormal eye movements, which over time mature into full-fledged paroxysms of torticollis.

Pattern of BPTI fits

The sudden attacks of head tilt are not preceded by any warning sign. It is the periodic painless spasm of the neck muscles that twists the neck, which is seen as an abnormal position of the head.

The "benign paroxysmal torticollis of infancy" typically presents in mornings. The head tilt may alternate from left to right in different episodes. Rarely it is accompanied by the lateral incurvation of the trunk, tortipelvis. In many cases 'changes in posture' and 'rise in body

Vestibular System of Inner Ear

Provides sense of balance and orientation of the position of the body in space.
The basis for smooth and well timed coordinated body movements.

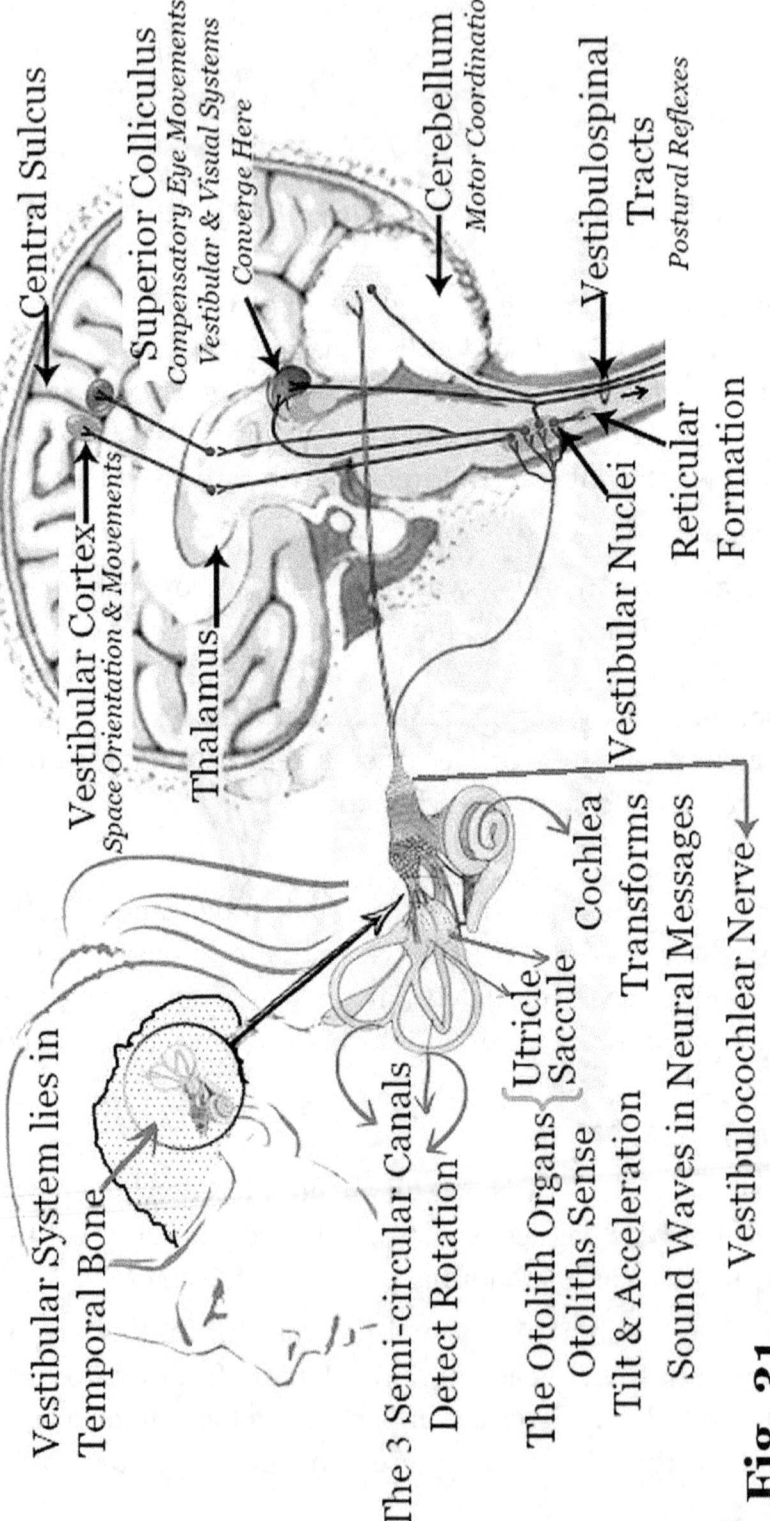

Central Sulcus

Superior Colliculus
Compensatory Eye Movements
Vestibular & Visual Systems
Converge Here

Cerebellum
Motor Coordination

Vestibulospinal
Tracts
Postural Reflexes

Vestibular Cortex
Space Orientation & Movements

Thalamus

Vestibular Nuclei

Reticular
Formation

Vestibular System lies in
Temporal Bone

The 3 Semi-circular Canals
Detect Rotation

The Otolith Organs { Utricle
Saccule
Otoliths Sense
Tilt & Acceleration

Cochlea
Transforms
Sound Waves in Neural Messages

Vestibulocochlear Nerve

Fig. 31

temperature' are noted to precipitate the attacks, but BPTI is also known to occur without any trigger.

Abnormal eye movements are the first to be noticed, followed by a lack of interest in the surroundings and drowsiness that ends in a still head tilt, which may persist through the sleep. Most of the attacks settle spontaneously within minutes, but some may persist for hours or days at a stretch.

The short-lasting episodes are more likely to mimic infantile fits. Especially because they are more often accompanied by symptoms of autonomic nervous system disturbance, such as nausea, vomiting, pallor, irritability, wobbliness, rotation of the eyes, incoordination, and occasionally spasm of limbs muscles. The inability to carry out voluntary movements effectively is more obvious after the first year of life. Around the same time, the head tilts become less prominent.

Outcome

On the whole, and despite prolonged and frequent spells that recur for years, the outcome is generally good. However, some of these children develop vertigo and/or migraine headaches during teens or early adulthood. History of migraine and/or motion sickness in an immediate family member of these infants is usual. *BPTI is therefore described as an age-dependent migraine-related disorder. Besides the genetic factor, it is believed to be vestibular system dysfunction (Fig. 31) caused by immaturity of central nervous system. Overall development of the affected children is normal.*

Medical evaluation is a must

No treatment is necessary for BPTI, but good clinical assessment of the cases is mandatory. It helps rule out treatable causes of torticollis. BPTI is a diagnosis of exclusion, wherein neurological examination, even in between the attacks, is normal. Nor is any abnormality detected on EEG or spine and brain imaging of these cases.

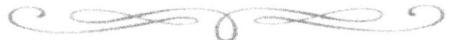

22. Sandifer's syndrome

Sandifer's syndrome was first described in 1962. It comprises of intermittent torticollis, spastic body movements, gastroesophageal reflux disease (GERD)*, and in a few, hiatus hernia**.

The cause

Though the precise underlying cause of this disorder is not yet determined, *the fitful abnormal posture is believed to be body's response to the pain caused by the passage of acidic contents of the stomach back into the food pipe.* This hypothesis is supported by the facts that the episodes are clearly associated with feeding, and most of the affected infants do not show any neurological abnormality. Nevertheless, subtle neurological abnormalities, such as poor eye contact and muscle stiffness, has been observed in some cases.

Clinical confusion

The triad of symptoms typically begins in infancy. *The early presenting symptoms like irritability, gurgling in throat, difficulty in swallowing and regurgitations get over-looked for habitual issues of the initial months of life, whereas the recurring breath holding spells, head till, upward deviation of the eyes, stiffening of the body, and writhing movements of the limbs are mistaken for infantile seizures.* As a result, and despite the fact that 1 in 5 parents seek professional help for regurgitation in their baby, Sandifer's syndrome is very rarely identified. Even then, the syndrome is reported to occur in up to 8% of gastroesophageal reflux disease cases. Boys are believed to be affected more frequently than the girls, but neither the male to female ratio nor the overall incidence of the disorder is known.

Consequences

Delay in the diagnosis results in an inappropriate management of this seizure-like activity. Although each episode generally lasts only for a couple of minutes, several of them occur in a day. As the time goes by they may adversely affect child's nutrition, growth, and development. Moreover, frequent silent refluxes lead to recurring inflammation and tissue damage in the food pipe. Some reflux material may even find its way into the windpipe, and from there down into the lungs. This results in bouts of spasmodic cough, periodic wheezing, difficulty in breathing, and recurrent pneumonia. These acute secondary issues grab the treating doctors' attention, which makes it difficult for them to clinch the underlying Sandifer's syndrome.

Medical evaluation and outcome

Infants and young children with torticollis, dystonic episodes, or atypical seizures should, therefore, be evaluated for GERD and Sandifer syndrome. Both GERD and Sandifer's syndrome are reactive attacks wherein expensive and comprehensive neurologic evaluation may not be necessary. *Early and appropriate management of these cases promises good results.*

----

*Gastroesophageal Reflux Disease (GERD): Fig. 32 pg. 92

** Hiatus Hernia: Fig. 33 pg. 93

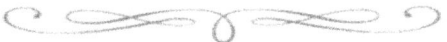

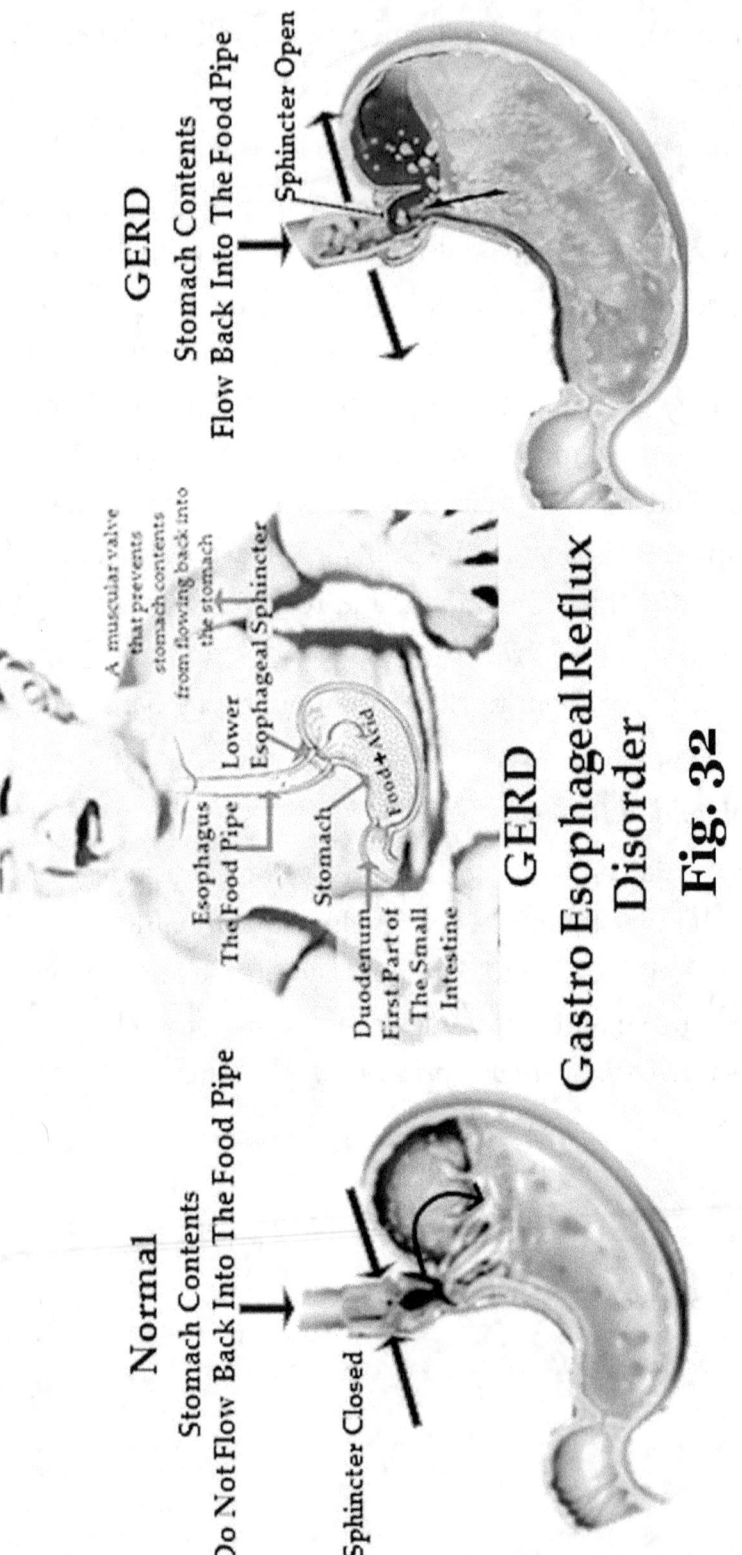

GERD

Gastro Esophageal Reflux Disorder

Fig. 32

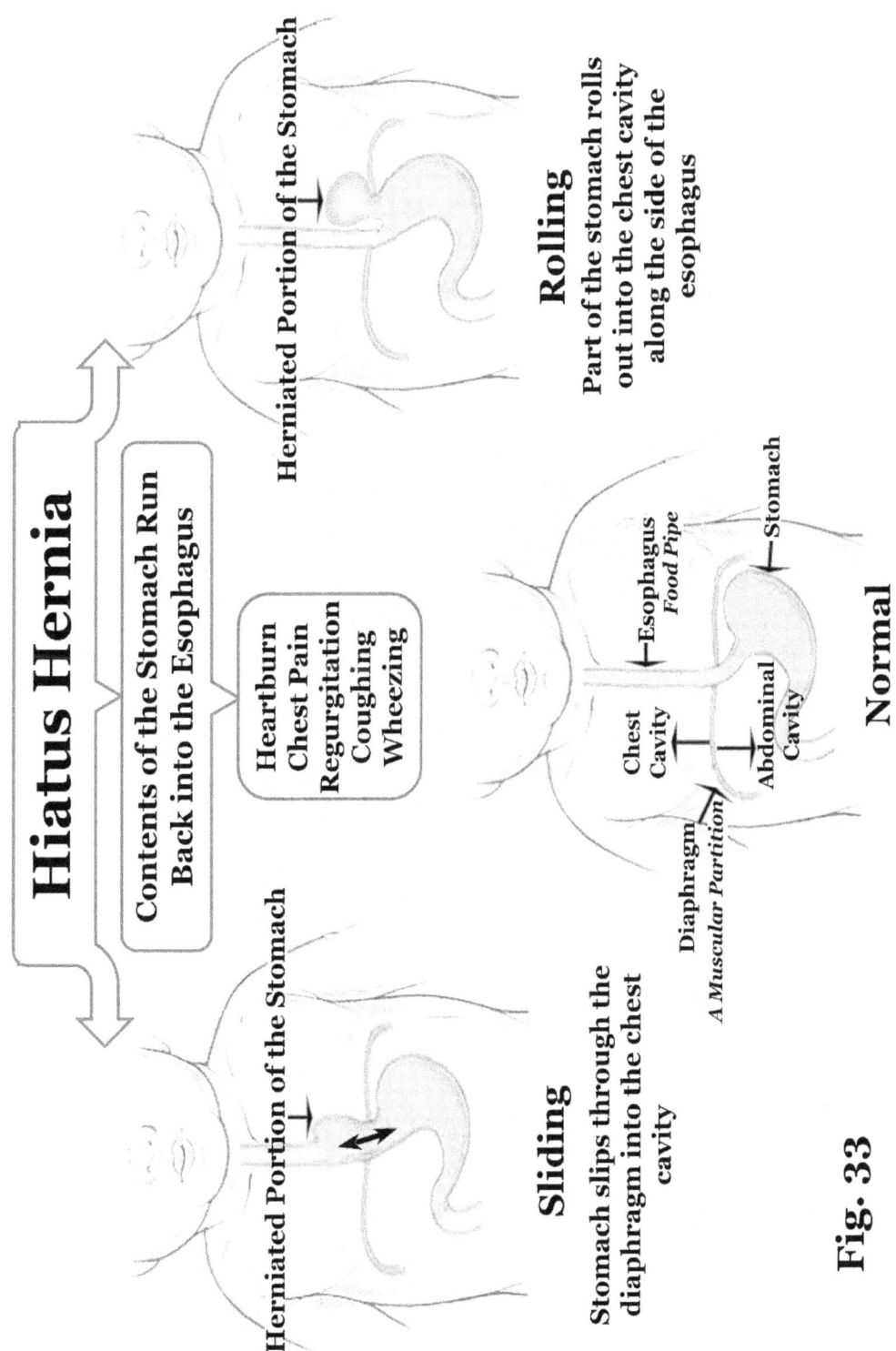

Hiatus Hernia

Contents of the Stomach Run Back into the Esophagus

Heartburn
Chest Pain
Regurgitation
Coughing
Wheezing

Herniated Portion of the Stomach

Rolling
Part of the stomach rolls out into the chest cavity along the side of the esophagus

Herniated Portion of the Stomach

Sliding
Stomach slips through the diaphragm into the chest cavity

←Esophagus
Food Pipe

←Stomach

Chest Cavity

Abdominal Cavity

Diaphragm
A Muscular Partition

Normal

Fig. 33

23. *Jerky Eye Movements: Nystagmus*

Periodic involuntary jerky movements of the eyes is a rare movement disorder of the eye muscles with the prevalence rate of about 1 in 700 infants. Of them, only 1 in 5 infants suffers from an underlying functional or structural abnormality of the cerebellum, midbrain, brainstem (Fig. 36) or anterior visual pathway*. These are classified as "acquired nystagmus". Rest fall in the category of "infantile nystagmus".

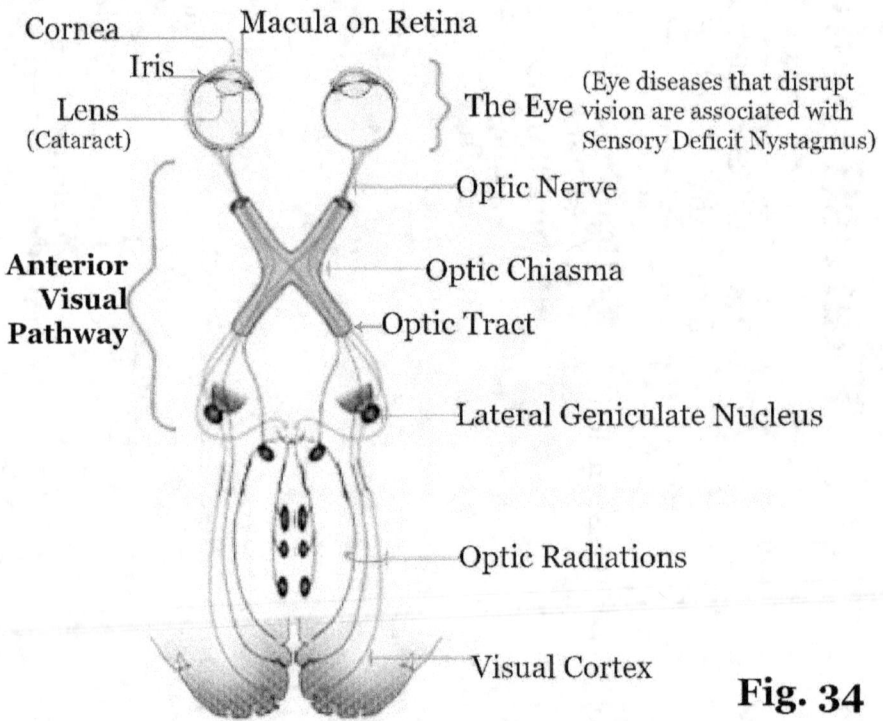

Cornea

Macula on Retina

Iris

Lens
(Cataract)

The Eye   (Eye diseases that disrupt vision are associated with Sensory Deficit Nystagmus)

Optic Nerve

Anterior Visual Pathway

Optic Chiasma

Optic Tract

Lateral Geniculate Nucleus

Optic Radiations

Visual Cortex

Fig. 34

Infantile nystagmus is broadly divided into idiopathic and sensory. Under "sensory nystagmus" are grouped inborn defects of the eyes that disrupt vision right from birth, and hence the development of movements of the eyes (Fig. 35). The nystagmus in Albinism, though usually listed separately, is also caused by early visual deprivation due

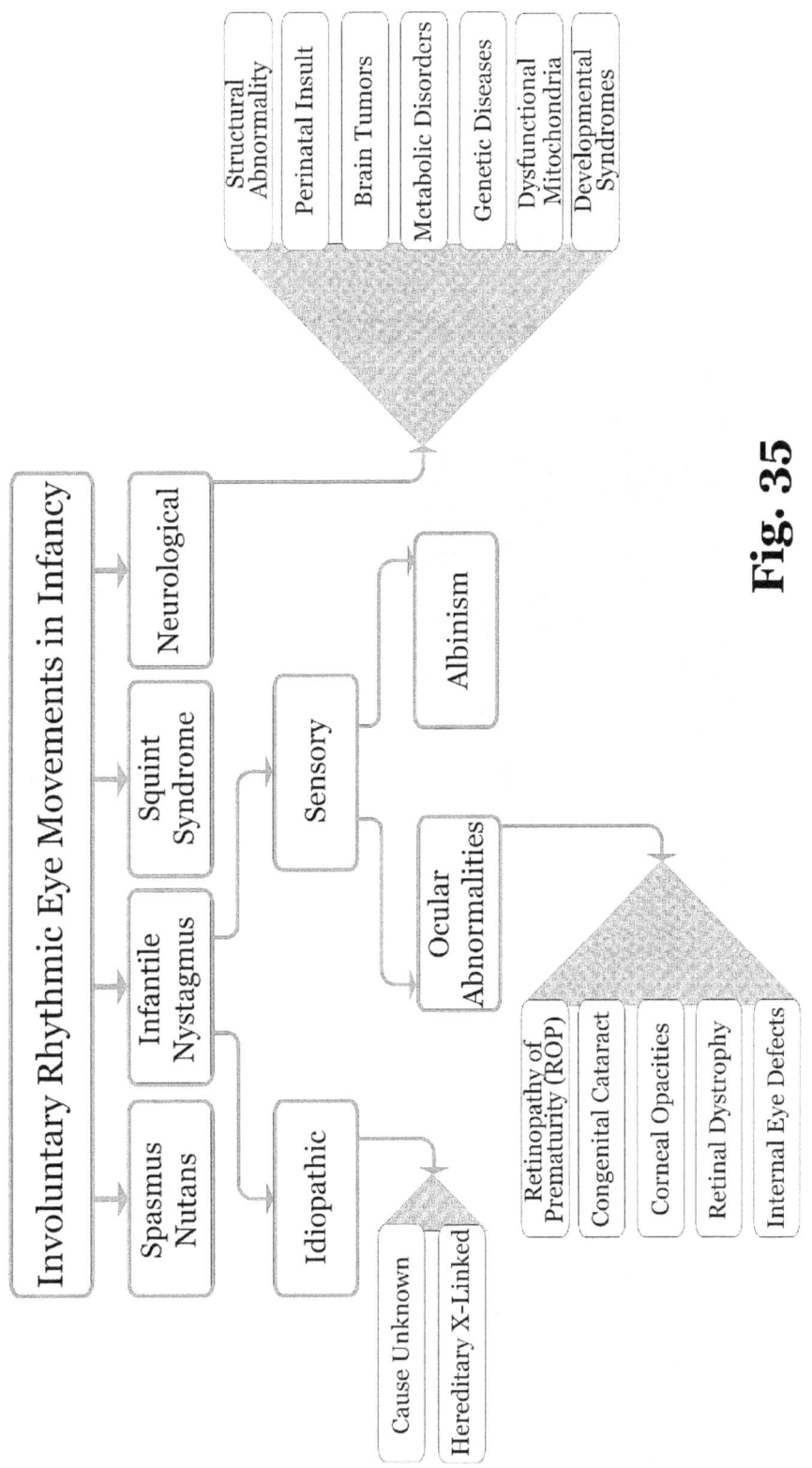

Fig. 35

to reduced colouring matter of the eye, in iris and retina, which is essential for clear vision.

The underlying cause of idiopathic infantile nystagmus, although often unknown, is present from birth, but the abnormal eye movements become apparent only around 6 weeks of age or soon thereafter when the baby begins to fixate objects. In comparison, the acquired nystagmus usually manifest in the latter half of infancy; Spasmus Nutans (pg. 99) being an exception with its onset between 4 and 36 months of age.

Mechanisms of nystagmus

In general, the mechanisms of nystagmus that is secondary to ocular and neurological abnormalities are better understood than those behind idiopathic infantile nystagmus. Numerous hypotheses have been proposed to explain this involuntary "to and fro" movements of the eyes in infants who have no visual pathway disease and no neurological abnormalities.

Idiopathic infantile nystagmus

Idiopathic infantile nystagmus is now believed to be due to a primary abnormality in the area of the brain responsible for the control of eye movements (Fig. 36). It has a familial predisposition. All possible modes of inheritance have been described. Sporadic cases are noted as well. However, the most common form is X-linked with mutations in FRMD7 gene. The expression of the disorder, both in FRMD7 and non-FRMD7 groups, varies in potency from person to person even within the same family.

Idiopathic infantile nystagmus usually persists for life, but in a small number of cases, it resolves spontaneously over few months. This is termed as "transient idiopathic nystagmus of infancy", and its underlying causes are grouped as follows:

1. Delayed Visual Maturation

Poor fixation of vision during first few weeks of life is a normal developmental phenomenon. Isolated delay in visual maturation can, therefore, offer a plausible explanation in these cases. This delay in development of visual control is neither associated with a defect in vision nor in the visual pathway, and the jerky eye movements resolve without treatment by 4–6 months of age.

2. Drugs

Several drugs, when taken during pregnancy, are known to cause nystagmus in the offspring. This applies to both, the controlled drugs prescribed during pregnancy for medical reasons like antidepressant Sertraline and anticonvulsants, and the recreational drugs like benzodiazepines, opiates, and cocaine. The nystagmus in these cases clears off completely on withdrawal of the drug, provided the teratogenicity** of the drug had not jeopardized the neurodevelopment of the baby in the womb.

3. Ocular motor control mechanism has adaptability to change

Eye movements mature during the first few weeks of life. But the muscles will work to focus an object only if there is reasonable visual input. Therefore the early elimination of the factors that adversely affect neural control, like vitamin B1 deficiency, congenital cataract etcetera, could reduce or eradicate nystagmus.

4. Subtle unknown events

Fight to focus

Despite the distressing eye-swings (from side to side, up and down, in a circular motion, or any combination of the three), the vision of infants with nystagmus remains blurred. They cannot clearly see the distance between the objects. Their ability to perceive the three dimensions of space is impaired. They are unable to balance over the stairs or through uneven surfaces. Their responses are therefore slow, clumsy and inconsistent.

Inconsistent behaviour is not a character trait of these children. The intensity of nystagmus is not consistent throughout the day. It worsens with tiredness, emotional stress, fear, effort to visualize, increased concentration, and in unfamiliar surroundings. In contrast, if a child is relaxed or sleeping the eye-swings are barely noticeable.

Reading, writing and the other skills of children with nystagmus are prejudiced by their fight to focus. Though intelligent, they are often looked upon as retarded, which hurts their intellectual, emotional and social well-being.

Children with acquired nystagmus suffer even more. They experience visual illusion in the form of constant movement of the surroundings. Their distress of nystagmus is compounded by the associated eye conditions in them, which requires detailed visual evaluation and imaging studies of the brain for precise diagnosis. Prompt assessment by an ophthalmologist is essential in all cases of nystagmus.

----

*Anterior Visual Pathway (Fig. 34): Refers to structures involved in vision before the Lateral Geniculate Nucleus, a relay center in the thalamus for the visual pathway. The posterior visual pathway refers to structures after this point.

** Teratogenicity: Ability to cause birth defects.

Macula (Fig. 34): Small area on the retina responsible for seeing in detail.

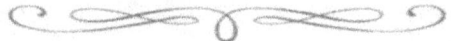

24. Head Nodding: Spasmus Nutans

Sudden attacks of involuntary, rapid and repetitive nodding of the head along with jerky movements of the eyes (nystagmus) is the characteristic clinical presentation of Spasmus Nutans, the Latin name for "nodding spasm". Head tilt, the third symptom during the episodes, is seen in less than half of the affected infants. No neurological or vision abnormalities are otherwise noted in these cases.

Incidence

Spasmus nutans is a rare paroxysmal movement disorder of infancy, which affects boys and girls equally. Its clinical presentation is not unique. Infantile nystagmus (Fig. 35), retinal diseases, brain tumors, and other potentially morbid neurologic diseases have the same symptoms. This creates a dilemma for the treating doctors. They hesitate to label the case an innocent disorder that would resolve spontaneously till the symptoms actually disappear. As a result, many cases are never reported, and the precise incidence remains open to debate.

The available records show that children of parents with social problems, financial insecurity, disturbed mental health, or with a history of alcohol or drug abuse are more frequently affected.

Cause

The exact underlying cause of this self-limiting benign condition is yet not clear. The affected infants are usually born small, which could either be due to premature birth or suboptimal weight gain during the fetal life. Some cases have a history of jitteriness in early infancy. These co-occurences may reflect a shared underlying mechanism.

Onset and progression

The triad of rapid eye movements head nodding and head tilt typically begins between 4 and 12 months of age. A few early and late onset cases (ranging anywhere between 2 weeks to 3 years of age) have been documented. Nodding and nystagmus are not equally prominent at the onset of the disorder, and the head tilt is not seen at all in almost half the cases. Head nodding resolves spontaneously by 4 years of age, but mild nystagmus may persist until puberty.

Head nodding

Periodic slow tremor like movements of the head is what first strikes concern in the parents. But the head nodding in Spasmus Nutans is not a movement disorder. It is believed to be the result of compensatory vestibule-ocular reflex to control the nystagmus, thereby improve the clarity of the vision. The nods, therefore, become conspicuous when the baby is engaged in an object of interest, and disappear when asleep.

The head usually moves at a lower frequency (2-3 Hertz*) than the nystagmus, in a gesture of "no-no". However, since the purpose of head nodding in these cases is to suppress nystagmus, the direction (yes-yes type or rotatory), and the range of head bob differ depending on the intensity, direction, and plane of eye-swings. Furthermore, some of these cases apparently use head-tilt to keep the nods of the head in an optimal path for the best possible visual perception.

Nystagmus

Nystagmus in Spasmus Nutans is typically fine high-frequency horizontal swings. In some cases, the swings may be vertical or torsional. It may affect one or both eyes. When in both eyes, the amplitude and/or phase of eye-swings in each eye differ. This disassociated movements of eyes makes it difficult to differentiate Spasmus Nutans, an innocent self-limiting disorder, from acquired nystagmus (Fig. 35) secondary to various brainpan lesions.

Nystagmus in one eye is often the presenting symptom of unilateral anterior visual-pathway disease or glioma**. In addition, some clinical conditions can occasionally resemble Spasmus Nutans. These include opsoclonus-myoclonus syndrome***, bobble-head doll syndrome****, infantile nystagmus, ocular motor apraxia*****, and so on. *Appropriate clinical evaluation along with a battery of tests are therefore absolutely essential to distinguish potentially morbid conditions from the innocent self-limiting clinical triad of nystagmus, nodding, and head-tilt.*

A diagnosis of exclusion

Besides the triad of symptoms, no eye or nervous system abnormality is found in cases of Spasmus Nutans. The results of neuroimaging, visual-evoked potential, and electroretinography studies are also normal in these cases.

Long term outcome

In spite of nystagmus during infancy, affected babies grow to have normal eyesight. However, about half of them develop squint, which may need surgical correction to overcome blurred vision. A few cases of mild developmental delay have also been reported in the literature, but in most the development of skills and mind are generally normal.

Regular medical checkups are a must

Evaluation at regular intervals by a professional is a must to keep track of the disease process until it actually disappears. And if any new neurological or developmental issues surface over the course of time, they too could be treated promptly and effectively.

What causes nystagmus in Spasmus Nutans?

Search for the precise cause of the nystagmus in Spasmus Nutans yet continues. Its disassociated nature suggests a defect in the cross connections of the nerves that synchronize the movements of the two eyeballs. This defect is supposedly in the midbrain at the level of the cranial nerves nuclei that control eyeball movements (Fig. 36).

However, the transient nature of this disorder indicates the possibility of delay in development of nerve connections. This explains why there is no typical pattern of nystagmus in cases of Spasmus Nutans. Genetic predisposition has also been considered because the disorder shows a tendency to be more frequent in some families.

Medications

Not necessary to control nodding and nystagmus of Spasmus Nutans.

Fig. 36

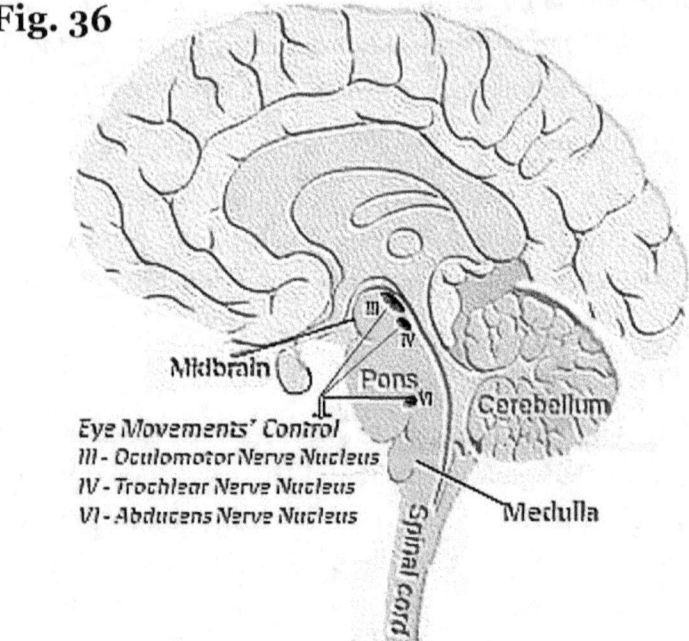

Midbrain

Pons

Cerebellum

Eye Movements' Control
III - Oculomotor Nerve Nucleus
IV - Trochlear Nerve Nucleus
VI - Abducens Nerve Nucleus

Spinal cord

Medulla

Midbrain, Pons & Medulla Form The Brain-stem

----

*Hertz: Cycles per second

Glioma: A malignant tumour of the glial tissue of the nervous system

***Opsoclonus-myoclonus syndrome: Also known as "dancing eyes, dancing feet syndrome". It mainly affects kids under 6 years of age. Rarely seen in infants under 6 months of age. It is an inflammatory neurological disorder secondary to underlying neoplastic disease, but not due to direct tissue invasion by the primary tumour or its metastases. The onset is usually abrupt, often severe, and it can become chronic. It is characterized by rapid, multi-directional eye movements, myoclonic jerks, sleep disturbances, poor speech, and irritability.

****Bobble-head doll syndrome: It is a rare neurological condition that typically presents in early childhood. It is characterized by head nodding in a gesture of yes-yes, which increases during walking and excitement, and decrease when the child is quiet, calm and engrossed in an activity. The exact cause of this disorder is not known. Cysts in the third ventricle of the brain are found in many affected children. These cysts are believed to cause an increase in water of the brain (cerebrospinal fluid), called hydrocephalus.

*****Ocular Motor Apraxia**: It is a rare self-limiting benign condition, wherein there is an inborn defect in control of voluntary, and purposeful eye movements. Consequently, rapid side-to-side eye movements, required to sustain gaze at a stationary object, are impaired. Instead, the associated abnormal jerky head movements enable the child to focus the desired object.

The jerky head movements are apparent at around 4 months of age when an infant has achieved reasonable head control. Prior to that, the inability to fixate on an object is commonly mistaken for blindness.

Fig. 37

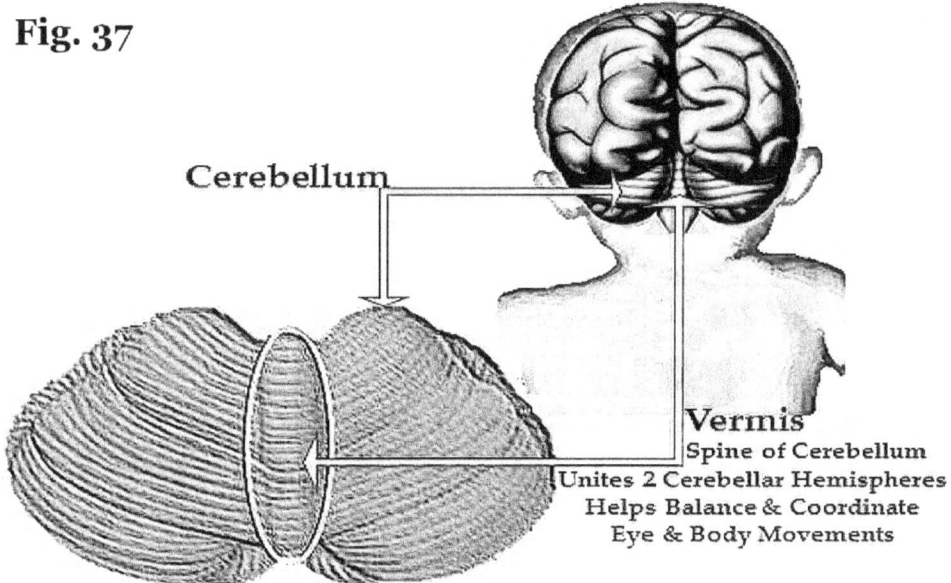

Cerebellum

Vermis
Spine of Cerebellum
Unites 2 Cerebellar Hemispheres
Helps Balance & Coordinate
Eye & Body Movements

The exact underlying cause of this disorder is not known. Underdeveloped cerebellar vermis has been found in some of the affected infants. No other neurological or extra neurological abnormalities are noted in these cases. Nevertheless, strabismus, developmental delay, and clumsiness have been reported in a small percentage of these cases.

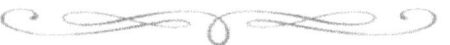

25. Benign Familial Infantile Epilepsy

Frequent fits in a 2-3 days old baby rock the boat, both of the parents and of the attending physician. Throughout the pregnancy and childbirth, nothing untoward or unusual happened. So now what? The doctor asks, "has anyone in the family had similar episodes"? "Yes, but he is fine now. Will she also be soon all right?", replies a confused concerned family member. Rather than fearing a battery of perinatal complications, a diligent family history could help identify the genetic cause for convulsions in such cases.

Cause, course, and incidence

Benign familial infantile epilepsy has a dominant mode of inheritance (Fig. 25). It commonly presents within the first week of life. Apparently frightening fits keep recurring for several months before resolving spontaneously, usually before the first birthday. The exact frequency of this disorder remains undetermined but is believed to be rare.

Outcome

This self-limited familial infantile convulsions are one of the few neonatal seizures that generally have a good outcome. They do not leave any ill effects on baby's development. However, in few cases continuation of periodic seizure activity later in life, developmental delay, and learning disabilities have been noted. These could be explained by genetic mutations that influence the likely course of the disorder.

Severity of seizures can alter the prognosis

The developing brain is very susceptible to seizures (pg. Neonatal Seizures Vs Jitteriness). For no apparent cause 15-20 convulsions per day jolt the tiny healthy body. The attacks are often quite severe and antiepileptic medications do not help. Yet the infants are remarkably normal in between the attacks. Status epilepticus is common in these cases.

The fits

Typically the fits are associated with behavioral arrest, eye deviation, tonic stiffening, and sometimes with myoclonic jerks. EEGs taken during the attack, show initial flattening followed by a bilateral spike and slow-wave discharges, often accompanied by a rhythmic clonic activity. Both partial or generalized seizures have been recorded.

But for diagnostic purposes, EEG is usually done in between the attacks, when no abnormality is detected on the recordings. MRI scan of the brain, and the blood work results are also within normal limits in these cases.

Diagnosis

The diagnosis of "benign familial infantile epilepsy" therefore rests on the family history of seizures in the newborn period. Two genes have been identified for this disorder, one on chromosome 20, and the other on chromosome 8. In a few cases, linkage to chromosomes 19, 16 and 12 have also been reported.

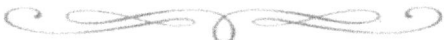

26. Fifth Day Fits

Parents are shattered by the sudden severe seizures in their 5 days old baby. They start groping for the cause.... Evil eye! Infection! Injury! Allergy! Witchcraft! Or ... what ...?

Nothing around the birth and thereafter indicated any abnormality in the baby. The doctor affirmed that he is a healthy full-term infant, and so was sent home on the third day of life. Then, what could have happened within two days of coming home?

Cause, course and incidence

Neonatal seizures often signal an underlying ominous neurological condition. But in cases of "fifth day fits" no cause is found, and the seizures keep occurring, at times 15 to 20 times per day. They stop as suddenly as they start; usually in a day or two, and definitely within 2 weeks. Once the fits stop, infants recover without any long-term consequences. This self-limiting disorder accounts for 5 to 7% of seizures in full-term infants.

Clinical picture

Clinically, the "fifth day fits" syndrome is quite distinct from other known causes of convulsions in newborns (Fig. 11). Those affected are healthy full-term babies born of an uncomplicated pregnancy and birth process. The onset of seizures is in the latter part of the first week of life; typically on the fifth day, which gives the name to this disorder.

The fits

The frequency of fits varies from case to case. In some, seizures recur every few minutes, whereas in others the interval between two attacks may be a couple of days. Most often it is multifocal jerking of the limbs or the face, of one side. The side on which it occurs usually fluctuates.

Temporary stoppage of breathing and cyanosis* are, at times, associated with the fits. The affected babies are frequently found to be jittery in between the attacks. Each convulsive episode lasts only for a few seconds to 3 minutes, but status epilepticus** is common, and may even last for days in a few.

Do anticonvulsant drugs help?

The common medications used to control convulsions seem to have no effect on infants with "fifth day fits" syndrome. Some studies link this syndrome to acute zinc deficiency. This is a "non-familial seizure disorder in neonates" for which no cause has been established.

----

*Cyanosis:** A bluish discoloration of the skin due to poor circulation or inadequate oxygenation of the blood

*Status Epilepticus:** Prolonged episodes of involuntary muscular contractions or frequent seizures that come occur close together and the person doesn't recover between seizures.

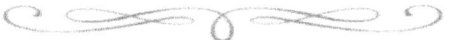

27. Alternating Hemiplegia

Alternating hemiplegia of childhood is predominantly an unpredictable neurodevelopmental syndrome*. It is very rare; the annual incidence is estimated at 0.9/100,000 newborns.

It manifests in early infancy, but not in the way as the name suggests. *Hemiplegia, the lack of ability to move one side of the body,* as the first symptom of the disease, is reported only by a few. In these cases, the earlier signs probably go unnoticed.

The earliest sign often gets overlooked

The first indicator of alternating hemiplegia is "recurrent episodes of abnormal eye movements". Almost all affected infants show nystagmus or single eye deviation, anytime between birth to 3 months of age. In most cases, the parents mark the asymmetry of the eye movements just when their baby begins to have eye contact. However, despite detailed medical examination and extensive investigations, no underlying abnormality for it is detected. Thus the earliest sign of this devastating disorder is mistakenly passed off as an innocent delay in the development of child's visual control, and the diagnosis gets delayed for a year or more.

Progression of the disability

Parents hope for the healthy development of their baby, which does occur but at a slow pace. Infants would have achieved only the very initial milestones when, at about 4 months of age, unprovoked attacks of muscular spasms and abnormal body posture begin. The recurrent attacks of flaccid alternating hemiplegia start shortly thereafter. Infants' level of consciousness is not disturbed by this disorder. Even during the attacks, babies are usually alert and responsive.

Each attack lasts anywhere from a few minutes to several days, and may affect one or both sides of the body. Those that involve both sides of the body are frequently associated with autonomic disturbances like fever, a change in colour (pallor or flushing), heart rate disturbances, and breathing difficulties (rapid breathing, wheezing, stridor or breath holding). These incapacitating paroxysmal phenomena remarkably disappear during sleep.

Besides these recurrent episodic events, the syndrome is characterized by persistent developmental delay, general learning disability, epileptic seizures, and choreoathetosis (irregular migrating contractions along with twisting and writhing movements). Consequently, the child has poor control on movements, which attributes to a number of clinical signs of the syndrome such as transient loss of eyeball movements, speech impediment, breathing difficulty, and drooling caused by an inability to swallow.

Alternating hemiplegia of childhood is a non-progressive and non-degenerative neurodevelopmental disorder. Its facets unfold as the infant grows; in most cases within the first 6 months of life, but may evolve any time from birth to teenage. The severity of the disease and its long-term effects differ considerably from case to case. This diversity in presentation and progression of the disease makes the diagnosis difficult. Nor is there any specific marker for the abnormality.

Genetic changes

Until recently the underlying cause for the syndrome was unclear. Genetic analysis has now shown it to be an autosomal dominant condition, but not necessarily inherited from the parents. Most affected infants do not have a positive family history of the disorder. More often than not, it is a new mutation. Nevertheless, a few cases of a parent to offspring transmission of the mutant gene have been documented.

Mutations in the ATP1A3 gene is believed to be the primary cause of alternating hemiplegia of childhood. This gene is expressed in nerve cells (Fig. 14) and contractile muscle cells of the heart. A single copy of the altered gene in each cell is sufficient to cause the disorder. Approximately 75% of cases show it. Others probably have one of the other mutations reported; CACNA1A (19p13), SLC1A3 (5p13) and ATP1A2 (1q21-q23).

Diagnosis is primarily clinical

The key to diagnosis are bouts of abnormal eye movements in the first 3 months of life, and the onset of recurrent dystonic or hemiplegic events in the first 6 months of life. For want of confirmation extensive investigations are done before labeling an infant a case of a severe neurodevelopmental disorder, which generally has an unrelenting course and poor outcome.

In cases of alternating hemiplegia, electrocardiogram (ECG) abnormalities are common but inconclusive, the nerve conduction studies and electromyography are ambiguous, and the biochemical analysis is usually within normal limits. On imaging, some cases show structural abnormalities of the brain but that too of unknown significance.

The clinical presentation and the resolution of the symptoms during sleep, however, indicate a central nervous disorder, which is emphasized by the expression of the causative gene in nerve cells. Though genetic testing can clinch the diagnosis, it is a time consuming specialized analysis, and is not always conclusive.

Nevertheless, investigations are essential to rule out other causes of neurodevelopmental disorder. The earlier the diagnosis, the more effective is the treatment, and minimum are the ill effects of alternating hemiplegia on child's development; attention deficit disorder, difficulties in acquiring speech, poor skills, and other behavioural problems.

----

*Syndrome: Medical condition characterized by a set of associated symptoms that consistently occur together. The word is derived from Greek word "dramein" that means to run, with the prefix "sun" which means together.

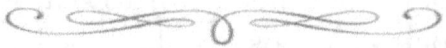

28. Neonatal Neurological Alarm Signals

Normal behaviour of infants is not well defined. Their expressions are confusing. Most are frequently fussy. Mingled in it are subtle signals of discomfort and potential indicators of serious diseases, which need to be identified promptly, and attended to accordingly. The challenge arises when one has to differentiate these 'alarm signs' from usual mood disturbance associated with social and emotional development. Therefore anything that feels is not quite right should be promptly brought to the attention of the paediatrician.

Infants below 6 months of age are particularly vulnerable to illnesses, both environmental and inborn. Infant behaviour that could be a sign of neurological disorder are:

1. Persistent irritability. An irritable infant is one who is agitated and cries with minimal stimulation and is unable to be soothed.

2. Difficulty in feeding

3. Persistent deviation of head and/or eyes

4. Persistent asymmetry in posture and movements

5. Persistently adducted thumbs in a fisted hand

6. Opisthotonos; spasm of the muscles causing backward arching of the head, neck, and spine

7. Persistent posture of flexed arms and extended legs

8. Lethargic infant, one who cannot maintain an alert state.

9. Apathy and immobility

10. Seeks attention infrequently

11. Floppiness, severe generalized hypotonia

12. Unusual body movements

13. Convulsions

14. Abnormal cry

15. The combination of setting-sun sign, vomiting, wide sutures and/or abnormal increase in skull circumference.

16. Breathing difficulties

17. Breath holding spells of longer than 20 seconds

18. Any change in a baby's behaviour as noticed by the parents.

19. Poor response to the smile of a caregiver.

20. Lacks eye contact

21. Any developmental delay noted by the parents

Very often, because of unsureness, parents opt to wait in the hope that with development the odd behaviour of their baby would disappear. 'Wait and see' perspective is a loss of the precious time. It delays identification of the defect, and thereby the necessary intervention. Early treatment can not only restrain the progression of the disorder but can also help in normal development. Infancy is the phase when the nervous system is still evolving. So, don't hesitate. Call your doctor and clear your doubts.

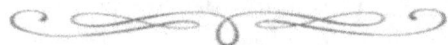

12. Unusual body movements

13. Convulsions

14. Abnormal cry

15. The combination of setting-sun sign, vomiting, wide sutures and/or abnormal increase in skull circumference.

16. Breathing difficulties

17. Breath holding spells of longer than 20 seconds

18. Any change in a baby's behaviour as noticed by the parents.

19. Poor response to the smile of a caregiver.

20. Lacks eye contact

21. Any developmental delay noted by the parents

Very often, because of unsureness, parents opt to wait in the hope that with development the odd behaviour of their baby would disappear. 'Wait and see' perspective is a loss of the precious time. It delays identification of the defect, and thereby the necessary intervention. Early treatment can not only restrain the progression of the disorder but can also help in normal development. Infancy is the phase when the nervous system is still evolving. So, don't hesitate. Call your doctor and clear your doubts.

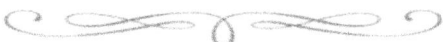

28. Neonatal Neurological Alarm Signals

Normal behaviour of infants is not well defined. Their expressions are confusing. Most are frequently fussy. Mingled in it are subtle signals of discomfort and potential indicators of serious diseases, which need to be identified promptly, and attended to accordingly. The challenge arises when one has to differentiate these 'alarm signs' from usual mood disturbance associated with social and emotional development. Therefore anything that feels is not quite right should be promptly brought to the attention of the paediatrician.

Infants below 6 months of age are particularly vulnerable to illnesses, both environmental and inborn. Infant behaviour that could be a sign of neurological disorder are:

1. Persistent irritability. An irritable infant is one who is agitated and cries with minimal stimulation and is unable to be soothed.

2. Difficulty in feeding

3. Persistent deviation of head and/or eyes

4. Persistent asymmetry in posture and movements

5. Persistently adducted thumbs in a fisted hand

6. Opisthotonos; spasm of the muscles causing backward arching of the head, neck, and spine

7. Persistent posture of flexed arms and extended legs

8. Lethargic infant, one who cannot maintain an alert state.

9. Apathy and immobility

10. Seeks attention infrequently

11. Floppiness, severe generalized hypotonia

Glossary

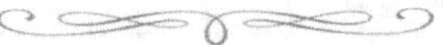

Glossary

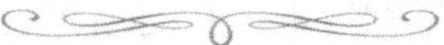

Bibliography

Agarwal M, Fox SM. Pediatric seizures. Emerg Med Clin N Am, 2013 Aug; 31(3):733–754 doi.org/10.1016/j.emc.2013.04.001

Alam S, Lux AL. Epilepsies in infancy. Arch Dis Child. 2012 Nov; 97(11):985-992. doi: 10.1136/archdischild-2011-301119.

American Academy of Pediatrics: Committee on Drugs. Neonatal drug withdrawal. Pediatrics. 1998; 101:1079–1088.

Anand KJ, Willson DF, et al. Tolerance and withdrawal from prolonged opioid use in critically ill children. Pediatrics. 2010 May; 125(5):e1208-1225. doi: 10.1542/peds.2009-0489.

Armentrout DC, Caple J. The jittery newborn. J Pediatr Health Care. 2001 May-Jun; 15(3):147-149. doi: 10.1067/mph.2001.114820

Auvin S, Pandit F, et al. Benign myoclonic epilepsy in infants: Electroclinical features and long-term follow-up of 34 patients, Epilepsia, 2006 Feb; 47(2):387–393. doi: 10.1111/j.1528-1167.2006.00433.x

Bakker MJ. et al (2006) Startle syndromes. Lancet Neurol. 2006 Jun; 5(6):513–524. doi: 10.1016/S1474-4422(06)70470-7

Berger A, Sharf B, Winter ST. Pronounced tremors in newborn infants: their meaning and prognostic significance. Clin Pediatr (Phila). 1975 Sep; 14(9) :834–835. doi: 10.1177/000992287501400908

Blackburn, S.T. Assessment and management of neurologic dysfunction. in: C. Kenner, J.W. Lott, A.A. Flandermeyer (Eds.) Comprehensive neonatal nursing: a physiologic perspective. WB Saunders, Philadelphia; 2013:564–607.

Bonnet C, Roubertie A, et al. Developmental and benign movement disorders in childhood. Mov Disord. 2010 Jul; 25(10):1317-1334. doi: 10.1002/mds.22944.

Bourgeois M, Aicardi J, Goutières F. Alternating hemiplegia of childhood. J Pediatr. 1993 May; 122(5 Pt 1):673-679. doi: 10.1016/S0022-3476(06)80003-X

Boylan GB, Stevenson NJ, Vanhatalo S. Monitoring neonatal seizures. Semin Fetal Neonatal Med. 2013 Aug; 18(4):202-208. doi: 10.1016/j.siny.2013.04.004.

Bradley's Neurology in Clinical Practice, 6th ed. 2012; Neurological Problems of the Newborn, Alan Hill Chap. 80:2111-2127

Brown RE, Basheer R, et al. Control of sleep and wakefulness. Physiol Rev. 2012 Jul; 92(3):1087-1187. doi: 10.1152/physrev.00032.2011

Calandra-Buonaura G, Alessandria M, et al. Hypnic jerks: neurophysiological characterization of a new motor pattern. Sleep Med. 2014 Jun; 15(6):725-727 doi: 10.1016/j.sleep.2014.01.024

Cambria S, Manganaro R, et al. Hyperexcitability syndrome in a newborn infant of chocoholic mother. Am J Perinatol. 2006 Oct; 23(7):421-422. doi: 10.1055/s-2006-951291

Caraballo RH, Capovilla G, et al. The spectrum of benign myoclonus of early infancy: Clinical and neurophysiologic features in 102 patients. Epilepsia. 2009 May; 50(5):1176-83. doi: 10.1111/j.1528-1167.2008.01994.x

Cerimagic D, Ivkic G, Bilic E. Neuroanatomical basis of Sandifer's syndrome: a new vagal reflex? Med Hypotheses. 2008; 70(5):957-61. doi: 10.1016/j.mehy.2007.09.011

Chen L. et al. Paroxysmal non-epileptic events in infants and toddlers: a phenomenologic analysis. Psychiatry Clin Neurosci. 2015; 69(6):351-359; doi: 10.1111/pcn. 12245

Chokroverty S, Bhat S, Gupta D. Intensified hypnic jerks: a polysomnographic and polymyographic analysis. Clin Neurophysiol. 2013 Aug; 30(4):403-10. doi: 10.1097/WNP.0b013e31829dde98.

Cilio MR. Review Article: EEG and the newborn. Journal of Pediatric Neurology 7 (2009) 25–43. doi: 10.3233/JPN-2009-0272

Cohen R, Shuper A, Straussberg R. Familial benign sleep myoclonus. Pediatr Neurol. 2007 May; 36(5):334–337. doi: 10.1016/j.pediatrneurol.2006.12.016

Cohen HA et al. Benign paroxysmal torticollis in infancy. Pediatr Neurol. 1993 Nov-Dec; 9(6):488-490

Cross JH. Differential diagnosis of epileptic seizures in infancy including the neonatal period. Semin Fetal Neonatal Med. 2013 Aug; 18(4):192-195. doi: 10.1016/j.siny.2013.04.003

Cross JH. Pitfalls in the diagnosis and differential diagnosis of epilepsy. Paediatrics and Child Health, 2009 May; 19(5)199–202 doi. 10.1016/j.paed.2009.02.003

Cuellar NG, Whisenant D, Stanton MP. Hypnic Jerks, a scoping literature review. Sleep Med Clin. 2015 Sep; 10(3):393-401 doi: 10.1016/j.jsmc.2015.05.010

Dalvi A. Pediatric tremor. Disease-a-Month. 2011 March; 57(3):160–165

doi: 10.1016/j.disamonth.2011.02.008

Danek A. Geniospasm: hereditary chin trembling. Mov Disord. 1993 Jul; 8(3):335-338. doi: 10.1002/mds.870080314

Deonna T, Martin D. Benign paroxysmal torticollis in infancy. Arch Dis Child. 1981 Dec; 56(12): 956–959.

Destee A, Cassim F, et al. Hereditary chin trembling or hereditary chin myoclonus? J Neurol Neurosurg Psychiatry. 1997 Dec; 63(6):804-7.

Deuschl G1. et al. The pathophysiology of tremor. Muscle Nerve. 2001 Jun; 24(6):716-735

Drigo P, et al. Benign paroxysmal torticollis of infancy. Brain Dev. 2000 May; 22(3):169-172 doi: 1016/S0387-7604(00)00099-1

Dubowitz LM, Dubowitz V, Morante A. Visual function in the newborn: a study of preterm and full-term infants. Brain Dev. 1980 Jan; 2(1):15-29

Dudek F Edward, Shao Li-Rong, Mossy Fiber. Sprouting and recurrent excitation: Direct Electrophysiologic Evidence and Potential Implications. Epilepsy Curr. 2004 Sep; 4(5): 184–187. doi: 10.1111/j.1535-7597.2004.04507.x

Einspieler C, et al. Human motor behavior: Prenatal Origin and Early Postnatal Development. Journal of Psychology 2008 Jan; 216(3):148–154 DOI 10.1027/0044-3409.216.3.148

Ehrt O. Infantile and acquired nystagmus in childhood. Eur J Paediatr Neurol. 2012 Nov; 16(6):567-572. doi: 10.1016/j.ejpn.2012.02.010.

Fanaroff and Martin's Neonatal-Perinatal Medicine, Vol. 2, 10th Edition 2014, Part II, The Central Nervous System: Chapter 58. Normal. and. Abnormal. Brain. Development. Pierre Gressens & Petra S. Hüppi - Chapter 62. Seizures in Neonates Mark S Scher

Ferrara J, Jankovic J.: Epidemiology and management of essential tremor in children; Paediatr Drugs. 2009 Oct; 11(5):293-307. doi: 10.2165/11316050-000000000-00000

Ferry PC. Shuddering spells. Seizure or not? Am J Dis Child. 1986 Jan; 140(1):19. doi:10.1001/archpedi.1986.02140150021022

Fons C, Campistol J, et al. Alternating hemiplegia of childhood: metabolic studies in the largest European series of patients. Eur J Paediatr Neurol. 2012 Jan; 16(1):10-4. doi: 10.1016/j.ejpn.2011.08.006.

Fransson P, Skiöld B, et al. Spontaneous brain activity in the newborn brain during natural sleep--an fMRI study in infants born at full term. Pediatr Res. 2009 Sep; 66(3):301-5. doi: 10.1203/PDR.0b013e3181b1bd84.

Fryer JC. Hypnic reflex: a spinal perspective. J Sleep Disord Ther. 2014 Nov; 3:177. doi:10.4172/2167-0277.1000177

Fusco L, Specchio N. Non-epileptic paroxysmal manifestations during sleep in infancy and childhood. Neurol Sci. 2005 Dec; 26 Suppl 3:s205-9. doi: 10.1007/s10072-005-0488-4

Fusco C, Valls-Solé J, et al. Electrophysiological approach to the study of essential tremor in children and adolescents. Dev Med Child Neurol. 2003 Sep; 45(9):624-7. doi: 10.1017/S0012162203001130

Futagi, Y, et al. Neurologic outcomes of infants with tremor within the first year of life. Pediatr Neurol. 1999 Aug; 21(2):557–561. doi: 10.1016/S0887-8994(99)00037-5

Futagi Y, Otani K, Goto M. Prognosis of infants with ankle clonus within the first year of life. Brain Dev. 1997 Jan; 19(1):50-54.

Giffin NJ, Benton S, Goadsby PJ. Benign paroxysmal torticollis of infancy: four new cases and linkage to CACNA1A mutation. Dev Med Child Neurol. 2002 Jul; 44(7):490-493 doi:10.1111/j.1469-8749.2002.tb00311.

Girard N, Raybaud C .Neonates with seizures: what to consider, how to image. Magn Reson Imaging Clin N Am. 2011 Nov; 19(4):685-708; vii. doi: 10.1016/j.mric.2011.08.003.

Good WV, Hou C, Carden SM. Transient, idiopathic nystagmus in infants. Dev Med & Child Neurol. 2003 May; 45 (5):304–307 doi: 10.1017/S0012162203000574

Gottlob I, Zubcov AA, et al. Head nodding is compensatory in Spasmus Nutans. Ophthalmology. 1992 Jul; 99(7):1024-1031.

Gottlob I, Wizov SS, Reinecke RD. Spasmus nutans: a long-term follow-up. Invest Ophthalmol Vis Sci. 1995 Dec; 36(13):2768-2771.

Hadjipanayis A, Efstathiou E, Neubauer D. Benign paroxysmal torticollis of infancy: an underdiagnosed condition. J Paediatr Child Health. 2015 Jul; 51(7):674-678 doi: 10.1111/jpc.12841

Hallberg B, Blennow M. Investigations for neonatal seizures. Semin Fetal Neonatal Med. 2013 Aug; 18(4):196-201. doi: 10.1016/j.siny.2013.03.001.

Heinzen EL, Swoboda KJ, et al. De novo mutations in ATP1A3 cause alternating hemiplegia of childhood. Nat Genet. 2012 Sep; 44 (9):1030–1034 doi:10.1038/ng.2358

Held-Egli K, Rüegger C, et al. Benign neonatal sleep myoclonus in newborn infants of opioid dependent mothers. Acta Paediatr. 2009 Jan; 98(1):69-73. doi: 10.1111/j.1651-2227.2008.01010.x.

Helen J. Differential diagnosis of epileptic seizures in infancy including the neonatal period. Seminars in Fetal & Neonatal Medicine, 2013 Aug.; 18(4):192–195. doi: 10.1016/j.siny.2013.04.003

Hill A. Neonatal seizures. Pediatrics in Review: 2000 April, 21(4)

Hoefnagel D, Biery B. Spasmus Nutans. Dev Med Child Neurol. 1968 Feb; 10(1):32–35. doi:10.1111/j.1469-8749.1968.tb02834.x

Huntsman RJ, Noel John Lowry NJ, Sankaran K. Nonepileptic motor phenomena in the neonate. Paediatr Child Health. 2008 Oct; 13(8): 680–684.

Jaberzadeh S, Brodin P, et al. Pulsatile control of the human masticatory muscles. J Physiol. 2003 Mar; 1; 547(Pt 2): 613–620. doi: 10.1113/jphysiol.2003.030221

Jackson L, Chandra V, Michie C. Hemivertebrae, are they always symptomatic? The West London Medical Journal. 2010; 2(3):5-12

Jaffer F, Avbersek A, et al. Faulty cardiac repolarization reserve in alternating hemiplegia of childhood broadens the phenotype. Brain. 2015 Oct; 138(Pt 10):2859-2874. doi: 10.1093/brain/awv243.

Jan MM. Shuddering attacks are not related to essential tremor. J Child Neurol. 2010 Jul; 25(7):881-883. doi: 10.1177/0883073809350222

Jankovic J, Madisetty J, Vuong KD. Essential tremor among children. Pediatrics. 2004 Nov; 114(5):1203-1205. doi: 10.1542/peds.2004-0031

Jayalakshmi P, Scott TF, et al. Infantile nystagmus: a prospective study of spasmus nutans, and congenital nystagmus and unclassified nystagmus of infancy. J Pediatr. 1970 Aug; 77(2):177–187.

Jensen FE. Neonatal Seizures: An update on mechanisms and management. Clin Perinatol. 2009 Dec; 36(4): 881. doi:10.1016/j.clp.2009.08.001.

Kabakus N, Kurt A. Sandifer Syndrome: a continuing problem of misdiagnosis. Pediatr Int. 2006 Dec; 48(6):622-5. doi: 10.1111/j.1442-200X.2006.02280.x

Kanazawa O. Shuddering attacks-report of four children. Pediatr Neurol. 2000 Nov; 23(5):421-4. doi: 10.1016/S0887-8994(00)00205-8

Keller S, Dure LS. Tremor in childhood. Semin Pediatr Neurol. 2009; 16:60–70 doi:10.1016/j.spen.2009.03.007

Kim JS, Park SH, Lee KW. Spasmus nutans and congenital ocular motor apraxia with cerebellar vermian hypoplasia. Arch Neurol. 2003 Nov; 60(11):1621-1624 doi:10.1001/archneur.60.11.1621

King RA, Nelson LB, Wagner RS. Spasmus nutans a benign clinical entity? Arch Ophthalmol. 1986 Oct; 104(10):1501-1504 doi:10.1001/archopht.1986.01050220095035

Kotagal P, Costa M, et al. Paroxysmal nonepileptic events in children and adolescents. Pediatrics 2002 Oct; 110(4); e46 doi: 10.1542/peds.110.4.e46

Kothare SV, Kaleyias J. Sleep and epilepsy in children and adolescents. Sleep Med. 2010 Aug; 11(7):674-85. doi: 10.1016/j.sleep.2010.01.012.

Kramer U, Nevo Y, Harel S. Jittery babies: a short-term follow-up. Brain Dev. 1994 Mar-Apr; 16(2):112-4.

Krägeloh I, Aicardi J. Alternating hemiplegia in infants: report of five cases. Dev Med Child Neurol. 1980 Dec; 22(6):784-91. doi:10.1111/j.1469-8749.1980.tb03746.x

Kryger MH, Roth T, Dement W. Principles and Practice of Sleep Medicine, 5th Ed.2011, PART II / Section 12 • Parasomnias

Lester BM, Bagner DM., et al. Infant neurobehavioral dysregulation: behavior problems in children with prenatal substance exposure. Pediatrics. 2009 Nov; 124(5): 1355–1362. doi:10.1542/peds.2008-2898.

Lester BM, Tronick EZ, et al. The maternal lifestyle study: effects of substance exposure during pregnancy on neurodevelopmental outcome in 1-month-old infants. Pediatrics. 2002 Dec; 110:1182–1192.

Levy M., Spino M. Neonatal withdrawal syndrome: associated drugs and pharmacologic management. Pharmacotherapy. 1993 May-Jun; 13(3):202–211. doi: 10.1002/j.1875-9114.1993.tb02725.x

Lewis GR, Pilcher R, Yemm R. The effect of stimulus strength on the jaw-jerk response in man. J Neurol Neurosurg Psychiatry. 1980 Aug; 43(8): 699–704.

Linda GM, van Rooij, et al. Treatment of neonatal seizure. Semin Fetal Neonatal Med.2013 Aug; 18(4):209–215 doi:10.1016/j.siny.2013.01.001

Linder N, Moser AM, et al. Suckling stimulation test for neonatal tremor. Archives of Disease in Childhood 1989 Jan; 64(1 Spec No):44–46

Lipson EH, Robertson WC Jr. Paroxysmal torticollis of infancy: familial occurrence. Am J Dis Child. 1978 Apr; 132(4):422–423.

Louis ED, Cubo E, et al. Tremor in school-aged children: a cross-sectional study of tremor in 819 boys and girls in Burgos, Spain. Neuroepidemiology. 2011; 37(2):90-95 doi: 10.1159/000330352.

Louis ED, Dure LS 4th, Pullman S. Essential tremor in childhood: a series of nineteen cases. Mov Disord. 2001 Sep; 16(5):921-3. doi: 10.1002/mds.1182

Malhotra RK, Avidan AY. Parasomnias and their mimics. Neurol Clin. 2012 Nov; 30(4):1067-1094. doi: 10.1016/j.ncl.2012.08.016.

Manni R. & Terzaghi M. Rhythmic movements during sleep: a physiological and pathological profile. Neurol Sci. 2005 Dec; 26(Suppl 3):181-185. doi: 10.1007/s10072-005-0484-8

Marchi LR, Seraphim EA, et al. Epileptic spasms without hypsarrhythmia in infancy and childhood: tonic spasms as a seizure type. Epileptic Disord. 2015 Jun; 17(2):188-93. doi: 10.1684/epd.2015.0738.

Mason AG, et al. Dissociation of nociceptive modulation of a human jaw reflex from the influence of stress. Exp Brain Res. 2007May; 182 (1):81-91. doi: 10.1007/s00221-007-0972-6

Maydell BV, Berenson F, et al. Benign myoclonus of early infancy: an imitator of West's syndrome. J Child Neurol. 2001 Feb; 16(2):109-12. doi: 10.1177/088307380101600208

Mayer G, Wilde-Frenz J, Kurella B. Sleep related rhythmic movement disorder revisited. J Sleep Res. 2007 Mar; 16(1):110-116. doi: 10.1111/j.1365-2869.2007.00577.x.

Méneret A, et al. PRRT2 mutations and paroxysmal disorders. Eur J Neurol. 2013 Jun; 20(6):872-878 doi: 10.1111/ene.12104

Mikati MA, Kramer U, et al. Alternating hemiplegia of childhood: clinical manifestations and long-term outcome. Pediatr Neurol. 2000 Aug; 23(2):134–141. doi: 10.1016/S0887-8994(00)00157-0

Mirmiran M, Maas YG, Ariagno RL. Development of fetal and neonatal sleep and circadian rhythms. Sleep Med Rev. 2003 Aug; 7(4):321-34. doi:10.1053/smrv.2002.0243

Montagna P. Sleep-related non epileptic motor disorders. J Neurol. 2004 Jul; 251(7):781-94. doi:10.1007/s00415-004-0478-0

Murphy WJ, Gellis SS. Torticollis with hiatus hernia in infancy. Sandifer syndrome. Am J Dis Child. 1977 Ma; 131(5):564-5 doi:10.1001/archpedi.1977.02120180078015

Myklebust BM, Gottlieb GL. Development of the stretch reflex in the newborn: reciprocal excitation and reflex irradiation. Child Dev. 1993 Aug; 64(4):1036-45.

Nabbout R, Soufflet C, Plouin P, Dulac O. Pyridoxine dependent epilepsy: a suggestive electroclinical pattern. Arch Dis Child Fetal Neonatal Ed. 1999 Sep; 81(2):F125-129. doi: 10.1136/fn.81.2.F125

Nardou R, Ferrari DC, Ben-Ari Y. Mechanisms and effects of seizures in the immature brain. Semin Fetal Neonatal Med. 2013 Aug; 18(4):175-84. doi: 10.1016/j.siny.2013.02.003.

Nelson Textbook of Pediatrics 19th ed. Part XXVII - The Nervous System – Chap.587: Conditions That Mimic Seizures. Mikati M & Obeid M. and Chap.586.7: Neonatal Seizures. Mikati M

Nunes ML, Jaderson Costa da Costa. Sleep and epilepsy in neonates. Sleep Medicine. 2010; 11(7):665–673. doi: 10.1016/j.sleep.2009.10.009

Orivoli S, Facini C, Pisani F. Paroxysmal nonepileptic motor phenomena in newborn. Brain Dev. 2015 Oct; 37(9):833-9. doi: 10.1016/j.braindev.2015.01.002

Pachatz C, Fusco L, Vigevano F. Benign myoclonus of early infancy. Epileptic Disord. 1999 Mar; 1(1):57-61.

Panagiotakaki E, Gobbi G, et al. Evidence of a non-progressive course of alternating hemiplegia of childhood: study of a large cohort of children and adults. Brain.2010; 133(Pt 12):3598–3610. doi: 10.1093/brain/awq295

Panagiotakaki E, De Grandis E, et al. Clinical profile of patients with ATP1A3 mutations in Alternating Hemiplegia of Childhood-a study of 155 patients. Orphanet J Rare Dis. 2015 Sep 26; 10:123. doi: 10.1186/s13023-015-0335-5.

Papageorgiou E, McLean RJ, Gottlob I. Nystagmus in childhood. Pediatr Neonatol. 2014 Oct; 55(5):341-51. doi: 10.1016/j.pedneo.2014.02.007.

Parker S, Zuckerman B, et al. Jitteriness in full-term neonates: prevalence and correlates. Pediatrics. 1990 Jan; 85(1):17–23.

Pavone P, Striano P, et al. Infantile spasms syndrome, West syndrome and related phenotypes: what we know in 2013. Brain Dev. 2014 Oct; 36(9):739-51. doi: 10.1016/j.braindev.2013.10.008.

Posner MI, Rothbart MK: Developing mechanisms of self-regulation. Development and Pschopatholog, 2000; 12(3):427-441

Pryor DS, Don N, Macourt DC. Fifth day fits: a syndrome of neonatal convulsions. Arch Dis Child. 1981 Oct; 56(10): 753–758.

Rennie & Roberton's Textbook of Neonatology, Chap.40, Neurological problems in neonates: 1065-1219

Resnick TJ, Moshe SL, et al. Benign neonatal sleep myoclonus. Relationship to sleep states. Arch Neurol 1986 March; 43(3):266-268. doi:10.1001/archneur.1986.00520030056014

Rosman NP, et al. The neurology of benign paroxysmal torticollis of infancy: report of 10 new cases and review of the literature. J Child Neurol. 2009 Feb; 24(2):155-60 doi: 10.1177/0883073808322338

Rosman, N.P., Donnelly, J.H., Braun, M.A. The jittery newborn and infant: a review. Developmental and Behavioral Pediatrics. 1984 Oct; 5(5):263–273.

Rothbart M., Ziaie H., O'Boyle C. (1992). Self-regulation and emotion in infancy. In N. Eisenberg & R. Fabes (Eds.), Emotion and its regulation in early development (pp. 7–23). San Francisco: Jossey-Bass.

Rothbart MK, Sheese BE, et al. Developing mechanisms of self-regulation in early life. Emotion review. 2011Apr; 3(2):207-213. doi:10.1177/1754073910387943.

Sander HW, Geisse H, Quintio C, et al. Sensory sleep starts. Journal of Neurology. Neurosurgery & Psychiatry 1998 May; 64(5):690. doi:10.1136/jnnp.64.5.690

Sarnat, H.B. Functions of the corticospinal and corticobulbar tracts in the human newborn. J Pediatr Neurol. 2003; 1(1):3–8.

Scagni P, et al. Benign paroxysmal torticollis of infancy: a case report. Minerva Pediatr. 2006 Oct; 58(5):499-501

Scher M: Diagnosis and Treatment of Neonatal Seizures, Chap. 8:109-137 Neurology: Neonatology Questions and Controversies by Jeffrey M. Perlman - 2012

Scher MS, Aso K, et al. Electrographic seizures in preterm and full-term neonates: Clinical correlates, associated brain lesions, and risk for neurologic sequelae. Pediatrics. 1993 Jan; 91(1):128-34.

Schmitt B, Baumgartner M, et al. Seizures and paroxysmal events: symptoms pointing to the diagnosis of pyridoxine-dependent epilepsy and pyridoxine phosphate oxidase deficiency. Dev Med Child Neurol. 2010 Jul; 52(7):e133-e142. doi: 10.1111/j.1469-8749.2010.03660.x.

Serino D, Fusco L. Epileptic hypnagogic jerks mimicking repetitive sleep starts. Sleep Med. 2015 Aug; 16(8):1014–1016. doi: 10.1016/j.sleep.2015.04.015

Sharieff G, Hendry P. Afebrile pediatric seizures. Emerg Med Clin North Am. 2011 Feb; 29(1):95-108. doi: 10.1016/j.emc.2010.08.009

Sheldon SH, Kryger MH, Ferber R. Principles and Practice of Pediatric Sleep Medicine, 2nd ed. 2014

Shimohira M, Iwakawa Y, Kohyama J. Rapid-eye-movement sleep in jittery infants, Early Hum Dev. 2002 Jan; 66(1):25-31. doi: 10.1016/S0378-3782(01)00232-8

Shuper A, Zalzberg, J, et al. Jitteriness beyond the neonatal period: a benign pattern of movement in infancy. J Child Neurol. 1991 Jul; 6(3):243–245. doi: 10.1177/088307389100600307

Silverstein FS, Jensen FE. Neonatal seizures. Annals of Neurology, Aug.2007; 62(2): 112–120. doi: 10.1002/ana.21167

Sims M., Artal R, et al. Neonatal jitteriness beyond the neonatal period: a benign pattern of unknown origin and circulating catecholamines. J Perinatal Med. 1986; 14:123–126.

Singer H, Mink J, Gilbert D, Jankovic J. Transient and Developmental Movement Disorders in Children: Paroxysmal Movement Disorders, and Hyperkinetic and Hypokinetic Movement Disorders; sec II, III & IV 70-257; Movement Disorders in Childhood, 2nd ed.2016

Smith DE, Fitzgerald K, Stass-Isern M, Cibis GW. Electroretinography is necessary for spasmus nutans diagnosis. Pediatr Neurol. 2000 Jul; 23 (1):33–36.

Snyder CH. Paroxysmal torticollis in infancy. A possible form of labyrinthitis. Am J Dis Child. 1969 Apr; 117(4):458–460.

Stern WM, Desikan M, et al. Spontaneously fluctuating motor cortex excitability in alternating hemiplegia of childhood: A transcranial magnetic stimulation study. PLoS One. 2016; 11(3): e0151667. Published online 2016 Mar 21. doi: 10.1371/journal.pone.0151667

Surtees R, Wolf N. Treatable neonatal epilepsy. 2007 Aug; Arch Dis Child. 92(8): 659–661. doi: 10.1136/adc.2007.116913

Swaiman's Pediatric Neurology: Principles and Practice 2012, 5th ed., Part IV Chap.16: Neonatal Seizures; Jensen FE, Silverstein FS.

Sweney M.T, Silver K, et al. Alternating hemiplegia of childhood: early characteristics and evolution of a neurodevelopmental syndrome. Pediatrics. 2009 Mar; 123(3):e534–e541. doi: 10.1542/peds.2008-2027

Thomas S, Proudlock FA, et al. Phenotypical characteristics of idiopathic infantile nystagmus with and without mutations in FRMD7. Brain 2008 May; 131(Pt 5):1259-1267. doi: 10.1093/brain/awn046.

Tibussek D, et al. Clinical reasoning: shuddering attacks in infancy. Neurology 2008 Mar; 70(13):38-41. doi: 10.1212/01.wnl.0000306698.75592.6e

Tinuper P, Provini F, et al. Movement disorders in sleep: guidelines for differentiating epileptic from non-epileptic motor phenomena arising from sleep. Sleep Med Rev. 2007 Aug; 11(4):255-267. doi: 10.1016/j.smrv.2007.01.001

Turanli G, Senbil N, Altunbasak S. Benign neonatal sleep myoclonus mimicking status epilepticus. J Child Neurol. 2004 Jan; 19(1):62–63. doi: 10.1177/08830738040190010708

Uria-Avellanal C, Marlow N, Rennie JM. Outcome following neonatal seizures. Semin Fetal Neonatal Med. 2013 Aug; 18(4):224-32. doi: 10.1016/j.siny.2013.01.002.

van Rooij LG, van den Broek, et al. Clinical management of seizures in newborns : diagnosis and treatment. Paediatr Drugs. 2013 Feb; 15(1):9-18. doi: 10.1007/s40272-012-0005-1.

Vasudevan C, Levene M. Epidemiology and aetiology of neonatal seizures. Semin Fetal Neonatal Med. 2013 Aug; 18(4):185-91. doi: 10.1016/j.siny.2013.05.008.

Vetrugno R, Montagna P. Sleep-to-wake transition movement disorders. Sleep Med. 2011 Dec; 12(Suppl 2):S11-S16. doi: 10.1016/j.sleep.2011.10.005

Ville D, Ginguene C, et al. Early diagnosis of pyridoxine-dependent epilepsy: video-EEG monitoring and biochemical and genetic investigation. 2013 Nov. Eur J Paediatr Neurol. 17(6):676-80. doi: 10.1016/j.ejpn.2013.06.005.

Volpe, Neurology of the Newborn, 5th ed. Philadelphia: Saunders Elsevier; 2008

Watkins RJ, Thomas MG, et al. The Role of FRMD7 in Idiopathic Infantile Nystagmus. J Ophthalmol. Volume 2012 (2012), Article ID 460956, 7 pages. doi: 10.1155/2012/460956.

Weinstein M, Marom R, et al. Neonatal neuropsychology: emerging relations of neonatal sensory-motor responses to white matter integrity. Neuropsychologia. 2014 Aug; 62(1):209-19. doi: 10.1016/j.neuropsychologia.2014.07.028.

Westenberger A, Max C, et al. Alternating hemiplegia of childhood as a new presentation of adenylate cyclase 5-mutation-associated disease: a report of two cases. J Pediatr. 2017 Feb; 181:306-308.e1. doi: 10.1016/j.jpeds.2016.10.079.

Wizov SS, Reinecke RD, et al. A comparative demographic and socioeconomic study of spasmus nutans and infantile nystagmus. Am J Ophthalmol. 2002 Feb; 133(2):256-62. doi: 10.1016/S0002-9394(01)01363-0

Yilmaz Ü, Serdaroglu A, et al. Childhood paroxysmal nonepileptic events. Epilepsy Behav. 2013 Apr; 27(1):124-129. doi: 10.1016/j.yebeh.2012.12.028.

Zupanc ML. Neonatal seizures. Pediatr Clin N Am 2004, 51:96

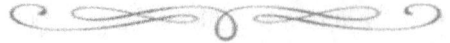

Author's Introduction

Seeing children through their health challenges is not only Renuka Chatterjee's profession but also her passion. She is a pediatrician with special interest in newborns, retired after more than 30 years of practice, of which for 20 years she worked as a neonatal intensivist.

The turmoil associated with parenting newborns is natural. Besides the ruffling due to the abrupt transition from intrauterine to extrauterine life, the needs of neonates are urgent, and often unclear. The subtle signals of their ill health keep parents on edge.

She has often sensed parents' anxiety and have managed to clear their doubts successfully, not only during clinical practice but also through her website.

The number of questions that pour in on this single topic is amazing. She answered many of them through http://www.childhealth-explanation.com/jitteriness.html and the related pages, yet a lot remained untold. Hence the book, "Jittery Baby and the Mimics of Fits in Early Infancy", which gives a deep insight into the normal and the abnormal causes of fits like activity that is commonly seen in little babies.

Do visit www.childhealth-explanation.com/meet-me.html to know more about Renuka. You can also post your concerns and get answers at "Ask Doc" or "Newborn Care Forum", the Free portals of the website, which she manages personally.

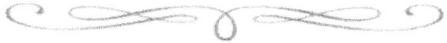

www.ingramcontent.com/pod-product-compliance
Lightning Source LLC
Chambersburg PA
CBHW081220280526
45787CB00006B/2459